REPTILE CLINICIAN'S HANDBOOK

A COMPACT CLINICAL AND SURGICAL REFERENCE

Fredric L. Frye, BSc, DVM, MSc, CBiol, FiBiol
Fellow, Royal Society of Medicine

KRIEGER PUBLISHING COMPANY
MALABAR, FLORIDA
1994

[Portions of this syllabus were abstracted from Frye, F. L. (1991). BIOMEDICAL AND SURGICAL ASPECTS OF CAPTIVE REPTILE HUSBANDRY, 2nd Ed., in two volumes and Frye, F. L. (1991) and A PRACTICAL GUIDE FOR FEEDING CAPTIVE REPTILES. Malabar, Florida; Krieger Publishing Company, Inc.

Original Edition 1994

Printed and Published by
KRIEGER PUBLISHING COMPANY
KRIEGER DRIVE
MALABAR, FLORIDA 32950

Copyright (c) 1994 by Krieger Publishing Company

All rights reserved. No part of this book may be reproduced in any form or by any means, electronic or mechanical, including information storage and retrieval systems without permission in writing from the publisher.
No liability is assumed with respect to the use of the information contained herein.
Printed in the United States of America.

> FROM A DECLARATION OF PRINCIPLES JOINTLY ADOPTED BY A COMMITTEE OF THE AMERICAN BAR ASSOCIATION AND A COMMITTEE OF PUBLISHERS:
> This publication is designed to provide accurate and authoritative information in regard to the subject matter covered. It is sold with the understanding that the publisher is not engaged in rendering legal, accounting, or other professional service. If legal advice or other expert assistance is required, the services of a competent professional person should be sought.

Library of Congress Cataloging-In-Publication Data

Frye, Fredric L.
    Reptile clinician's handboook: a compact clinical and surgical reference/ Fredric L. Frye.
      p.   cm.
    Includes index.
    ISBN 0-89464-783-0 (alk. paper)
    1. Captive reptiles—Diseases. 2. Captive reptiles—Surgery. 3. Captive reptiles. 4. Veterinary clinical pathology. I. Title.
SF997.5.R4F78   1994
639.3'9—dc20
                                            92-23869
                                                  CIP

10 9 8 7 6 5 4 3 2

DEDICATION

To Brucye, Lorraine, Erik, Bice, Noah, and Ian.

To the memory of my parents whose forebearance during my childhood made it possible for me to pursue what began as a hobby, and soon became my life's calling.

To the memory of my late father-in-law, Arnold, who probably thought my interests in reptiles were thoroughly weird, but always seemed genuinely fascinated by what I was doing with my scaly patients.

ACKNOWLEDGMENTS

As with my other writing projects, the first eyes other than mine to see the manuscripts have been those of my wife of more than thirty-seven years, Brucye, who as my most severe critic, has shown much perspicacity in her editing. Her dedication and friendship have been truly inspirational.

I am indebted to the entire production staff of my publisher, Krieger Publishing Co., Inc. for their expertise, enthusiasm, and support for my efforts to create "user-friendly" reference texts in the subjects to which I have devoted most of my professional career. Each of the book projects of mine that they have published has been a pleasure to see through to completion. For her editorial skills, I am especially grateful to Elaine Rudd, whose constructively critical suggestions were always right on the mark.

CONTENTS

Acknowledgments	iv
List of Tables	viii
Introduction	xi

CHAPTER 1
GENERAL CONSIDERATIONS — 1
   A Brief Description of Reptiles — 1
   Environmental Considerations Related to Captivity — 7

CHAPTER 2
NUTRITION — 10
   Provision of an Adequate Water Supply — 13
   Selection of Food — 14
   Apprehension of Prey and Gathering of Fodder — 20
   Initial Processing — 23
   Assimilation — 25
   Elimination — 27
   Miscellaneous Factors and Their Effects on Nutrition — 28

CHAPTER 3
CLINICAL LABORATORY SAMPLE COLLECTION AND PROCESSING — 70
   Skin — 72
   Blood — 73
   Bone Marrow — 79
   Staining — 80
   Urine — 83
   Feces — 85

Gastric Lavage Specimens	86
Sputum	87
Semen	88
Microbiological Sampling	89
Cerebrospinal Fluid	91
Tissues	91
Stomach, Intestinal Contents and Water for Toxicology	96
Tracheal and Transtracheal Specimens	96
Specimens for Parasitological Identification	97
Additional Tips	98
Appendix	100

CHAPTER 4
CLINICAL METHODS

	133
Obtaining an Adequate History	133
Physical Restraint and Transport	133
The Use of Induced Vago-Vagal Response for Short-Term Restraint	138
Chemical Restraint/Anesthesia	138
Preanesthetic Parasympatholytic Medication	139
Tranquilizers	140
Local, Line, and Block Anesthesia	140
Euthanasia	141
Physical Examination	141
Fluid Replacement and Maintenance Therapy	151
Blood Transfusion	152
Obtaining Diagnostic Material from the Respiratory Tract	153
Obtaining Diagnostic Material from the Caudal Alimentary Tract	154

CHAPTER 5
SOME PRACTICAL SURGICAL AND NON-SURGICAL PROCEDURES — 160

- Anesthesia — 161
- Fractures — 161
- Gastrotomy and Enterotomy — 162
- Prolapses — 162
- Salpingotomy/Caesarian Delivery — 164
- Orbital Enucleation — 164
- Incision and Repair of the Chelonian Shell — 165
- Application of Epoxy Resin-Impregnated Fiberglass Patches — 167
- Amputations — 171
- Cryosurgery — 171
- Radiofrequency Electrosurgery — 172
- Repair of Maxillofacial and Mandibular Fractures — 173
- Overgrown Mouthparts and Claws — 176
- Sutureless Treatment of Skin Lacerations and Abrasions — 176
- Nonsurgical Retrieval of Gastric Foreign Bodies — 177
- Dystocia — 179
- Special Bandaging Techniques — 180
- Treatment Methods — 181
- Egg Incubation Methods — 182

Appendix A Reptile Information Forms — 209
Appendix B Lists of Nontoxic and Toxic Plants — 219
Appendix C Species List Cross-Referenced by Common Name — 230
Appendix D Species List Cross-Referenced by Scientific Name — 248
Index — 266

LIST OF TABLES

Food Preferences for Selected Snake Species	30
Food Preferences for Selected Lizard Species	44
Food Preferences for Selected Turtles, Terrapins, and Tortoises	53
Food Preferences for Crocodilians	61
Food Preferences of the Tuatara	62
Common Nutritious Plants	63
Food Values	66
Number of Erythrocytes Per Cubic Milliliter of Blood in Reptiles	104
Leukocytic Formulae of Various South African Reptiles	108
Range of Frequencies of the Different Types of Leukocytes Throughout the Year in Reptiles	110
Seasonal Changes in the Leukocytic Frequencies of Reptiles	111
Plasma Electrolytes	112
Packed Cell Volume and Certain Organic Constituents of Blood	119
Summary of Reptilian Blood Cell Histochemistry	128
Summary of Reptilian Granulocytes and Monocytes	131
Electrophysical Characteristics of Two Ultrasonic Dopplers	155
Chemical Restraint and Anesthetic Agents	156
Parenteral and Oral Antibiotics Used in Reptiles	183
Miscellaneous Drugs Used in Captive Reptiles	189
Topical Ointments, Sprays, and Solutions Used on Reptiles	195

REPTILE CLINICIAN'S HANDBOOK

Wound-Irrigating Solutions	196
Parasiticides	197
Metric/English/Apothecary Conversion Values	204
Kg/M^2/lb Conversions	206
Temperature Conversion	207

BOOKS BY THE AUTHOR

HUSBANDRY, MEDICINE AND SURGERY IN CAPTIVE REPTILES

BIOMEDICAL AND SURGICAL ASPECTS OF CAPTIVE REPTILE HUSBANDRY

PHYLLIS, PHALLUS, GENGHIS COHEN & OTHER CREATURES I HAVE KNOWN

FIRST AID FOR YOUR DOG

FIRST AID FOR YOUR CAT

SCHNAUZERS, A COMPLETE OWNER'S MANUAL

MUTTS, A COMPLETE OWNER'S MANUAL (simultaneously published in the United Kingdom as MONGRELS, A COMPLETE OWNER'S MANUAL)

BIOMEDICAL AND SURGICAL ASPECTS OF CAPTIVE REPTILE HUSBANDRY, 2nd Ed.

A PRACTICAL GUIDE FOR FEEDING CAPTIVE REPTILES

CAPTIVE INVERTEBRATES: A GUIDE TO THEIR BIOLOGY AND HUSBANDRY

IGUANAS: A GUIDE TO THEIR BIOLOGY AND CAPTIVE CARE

INTRODUCTION

The increasing interest in reptiles as subjects for public display, biomedical research, biology education, production of high quality protein human food converted from nonhuman food sources, and for a renewable source of valuable leather has presented veterinary clinicians with an opportunity to broaden their skills. Concomitant with this opportunity is the necessity to become familiar with the special techniques by which these animals may be handled safely and effectively.

Shortly after the publication of the second edition of my BIOMEDICAL AND SURGICAL ASPECTS OF CAPTIVE REPTILE HUSBANDRY, requests were received from veterinary practitioners for a brief and "user-friendly" syllabus and drug formulary for instant reference. What follows is a compendium that was abstracted and compiled from two of my recent publications and experiences gained over a quarter century of active private and institutional practice. The interested reader is encouraged to obtain the references to the original publications cited in this syllabus in the two-volume text and feeding guide noted above. Illustrative materials have been omitted in order to keep the cost of producing this syllabus as modest as possible.

CHAPTER 1

GENERAL CONSIDERATIONS

Reptiles are air-breathing creatures who reproduce by internal fertilization. The reptilian egg is similar to its avian counterpart; the embryonic membranes include an amnion, chorion, allantois (or chorioallantois), but an air chamber is lacking. The young are not larval but, rather, are miniatures of their parents. Some reptiles, particularly many lizards and a few snakes, are parthenogenetic; others display polyploidy as a normal complement of their chromosomal endowment. Yet others have their sex determined by the temperature at which their eggs are incubated. Unlike the popular belief, reptiles do not possess slimy skin, their tongues cannot sting, and when decapitated, they do not wait until dusk to die. In summary, these animals have enjoyed a remarkable success in exploiting their environments and surviving since the Mesozoic era long before prosimian primates evolved from tree shrews. Were it not for the destruction of their habitats by some of humankind's less noble endeavors, reptiles surely would be enjoying even more success in pursuit of their livelihoods.

A BRIEF DESCRIPTION OF REPTILES

The Class Reptilia consists of four orders:
CHELONIA: the turtles, tortoises, and terrapins
This order contains approximately 400 species. These

creatures possess four limbs and their ribs and vertebrae are contiguous and attached to a bony (or in some species, a leathery) shell; the upper, often high-domed portion is called the "carapace" and the lower, flattened portion which covers the belly, is called the "plastron." Unlike other vertebrates, the chelonian scapulae lie *beneath* the ribs, rather than on top of them. All Chelonians are oviparous, or egg-laying. The male possesses a single penis and often has a concave plastron which helps accommodate the often highly convex curvature of the caudal portion of the female's carapace. Others, especially the aquatic and semiaquatic turtles and terrapins, are more flattened when viewed from the side. They inhabit most temperate and tropical regions of the earth. Some of these animals hibernate or, more accurately, *brumate*; many others do not. These nonhibernating species should not be placed into artificial hibernation. Although most reptiles are termed "poikilothermic" with body temperatures influenced by their surrounding or ambient temperatures, some appear to be at least partially endothermic. This endothermicity is best represented by leatherback sea turtles, some brooding female pythons, and a few of the largest monitor lizards. The internal heat production is believed to originate from digestive and other metabolic processes in the first instance, and other mechanisms in the others. The deep-core temperatures of these turtles can be significantly warmer than the surrounding sea water—which may be quite cold in northern latitudes.

CROCODILIA: the alligators, crocodiles, caiman, and gavials (gharials)

There are 23 species extant, although at one time, many more species existed. These quadripedal, generally robust creatures are partial to aquatic environments in tropical and subtropical portions of the world, and are only rarely found far from bodies of water. Some are partially marine and are often found miles from the nearest land mass. The crocodilians are characterized physically by their osteoderm-plated integument, functional four-chambered heart, well developed hard palate that separates the oral cavity from the nasal passages, closeable eyelids fitted with transparent nictitating membranes, valvular eliptical nostrils and ear slits, powerful tail, prominent teeth, and the manner in which the fourth lower teeth fit into their upper jaw: in the true crocodiles and gharials, these teeth fit into a shallow groove-like depression in the labial edge of the upper jaws; in the alligators and caiman, these fourth lower teeth fit into conical pits in the upper jaw. Therefore, when viewing a crocodile or a gharial with its mouth closed from the side, the fourth lower teeth can be seen; these teeth are screened from view in the alligators and caimans. All of the crocodilians are oviparous. The males possess a single penis. The female crocodilians construct nests consisting of decaying vegetable matter which, as it decomposes, produces the warmth necessary for incubation.

Like many of the lizards and some chelonians, the sex of the embryos is at least partially, if not entirely, determined by the temperature at which the eggs are incubated. These nests are carefully tended by one or both parents and when the eggs begin to hatch, the hatchlings are aided in freeing themselves from their confining eggshells and may be carried to the nearest body of water. Parental care may continue for up to three years.

SQUAMATA: the scaled reptiles

This order is divided into two main suborders, one of which is further subdivided into a single small family.

Suborder **SAURIA**: these are the lizards of which approximately 3,000 species in 22 families are known. Some of these creatures possess two pairs of limbs; others have only a pair (forelimbs); yet others lack limbs entirely. Most lizards have moveable eyelids, external auditory canals covered by tympanic membranes; others are more snake-like and lack eyelids; others do not possess external ear drums. Some lizards are egg-laying; others retain the eggs in the body of the female until it is time for them to "hatch"; this form of reproductive strategy is termed "ovoviviparity" and the egg "shell" is little more than a membranous covering. The male lizards possess twin penile organs, called "hemipenes." Lizards have been remarkably successful in exploiting a wide variety of environments and habitats ranging from tropical to temperate to desert to alpine to marine aquatic. A group of snake-like or worm-like creatures have been subdivided into the family Amphisbaenidae. Only four venomous species of lizards exist, comprising members of a single family, Helodermatidae, and a solitary genus, *Heloderma*. All are found in the southwestern United States, Mexico, and northernmost Central America. Depending upon their family, lizards have integuments that are smooth; others are heavily and roughly keeled and/or spiky; yet others have either exquisitely soft, hobnail-like, or plated textures.

Suborder **SERPENTES**: these are the true snakes, limbless creatures that are believed to have descended from lizard ancestors. There are 12 families and approximately 2,700 species of snakes extant. Snakes have successfully exploited a wide range of habitats and environments inhabiting tropical, temperate, desert, marine and fresh water aquatic. Snakes differ in size from the tiny worm and sharp-tailed snakes barely a dozen centimeters in length, to the giant pythons, boas and anacondas, some of which may grow to more than 7 meters and can weigh over 150 kilograms. Some snakes are terrestrial; others are arboreal; yet others are strictly aquatic and can barely move on solid surfaces. All snakes lack moveable eyelids and external ears; instead, their eyes are covered by a transparent tertiary shield-like spectacle which is a derivative of the integument and is shed and renewed each time the animal molts its skin. In texture, the skin may be smooth and shiny, heavily keeled, or tubercular. Like their lizard cousins, there are both egg-laying and live-bearing snakes. As in the lizards, the males possess a pair of hemipenes. Many snakes possess venom and venom delivery systems; some secrete potent and lethally virulent venoms injected through hollow fangs located in the front of the mouth, either fixed in place or hinged so that they are deployed only when the mouth is opened; others are rear-fanged; most, but not all of these, are harmless to humans; still others can inflict severe envenomation. Some subdue their living prey by throwing one or more constricting coils about the animal and applying sufficient pressure to induce asphyxia. The prey is not, contrary to popular belief, crushed. As noted in the brief description of the chelonians, most reptiles are strictly hetero- or poikilothermic; another exception to this condition are some brooding female pythons who, after depositing their eggs, coil about their clutches and periodically contract their skeletal muscles. These rhythmic muscular twitches produce endothermic heat which aids in the incubation process of the developing embryos.

RHYNCHOCEPHALIA: the tuatara

This order is occupied by a single genus and perhaps only one or two species; this matter is in some dispute presently.

The tuatara, superficially a lizard-like creature, bears a resemblance to an iguana. However, because of its anatomical morphology, is classed in an order of its own. Often called a "living fossil," the tuatara is a relic creature which is found on a few islands offshore from New Zealand where it shares dank burrows with petrels and cockroaches upon which it feeds. Because of its rarity, only accredited—and highly fortunate—zoological collections have been granted access to one or more tuataras.

The tuatara lays eggs and these require more than a year of incubation at relatively low temperatures to hatch. The male tuatara lacks an erectile penis; during copulation, the male and female appose their cloacal vents and semen is instilled into the cloaca and terminal reproductive tract of the female.

Within the clinical setting, it is helpful to be able to identify reptiles—at least with respect to their family, if not their genus and species. One of the questions asked most frequently by my colleagues is, "What books do you recommend to help me learn to recognize and differentiate one snake, lizard, turtle, tortoise, or crocodilian from another?" Not only can such information help convey a sense of confidence of one's clinical abilities in your reptile-owning clients, but it can possibly be truly life-saving when encountering a snake that might be venomous or hazardous to you and your staff.

With that question in mind, of particular value are Ernst and Barbour's TURTLES OF THE WORLD; Goin and Goin's INTRODUCTION TO HERPETOLOGY; Grenard's HANDBOOK OF ALLIGATORS AND CROCODILES; Grzimek's ANIMAL LIFE ENCYCLOPEDIA, Vol. 6, Reptiles; Burghardt and

Rand's IGUANAS OF THE WORLD: THEIR BEHAVIOR, ECOLOGY AND CONSERVATION; Martin's MASTERS OF DISGUISE: A NATURAL HISTORY OF CHAMELEONS; Mehrtens' LIVING SNAKES OF THE WORLD IN COLOR; Peters' DICTIONARY OF HERPETOLOGY; Porter's HERPETOLOGY; Ross's CROCODILES AND ALLIGATORS; and Staniszewski's THE MANUAL OF SNAKES AND LIZARDS. In addition, one should have a copy of Life Nature Library's REPTILES. Most of these texts are available from used book dealers specializing in herpetology and/or natural history literature.

ENVIRONMENTAL CONSIDERATIONS RELATED TO CAPTIVITY

As noted above, reptiles can be partially characterized by their habits: some are aquatic or semiaquatic, arboreal, or terrestrial. The latter grouping can be further divided into those that live on the surface of the soil; those that are fossorial or burrowing; and lastly, those that are thigmotactic, or prefer to wedge themselves into rocky crevices when they are not thermoregulating by basking in the sunlight. Some reptiles are strictly diurnal and are only found during daylight hours. Others are strictly nocturnal, coming out after sundown. Yet others are termed "crepuscular" and are active during dusk or just before dawn.

In order to maintain healthy reptiles in captivity, it is essential to match their optimal environment as closely as possible. When kept in overly moist conditions, terrestrial forms often develop dermatitis or other integumentary disorders; aquatic species kept in dry habitats may become dehydrated because they are unable or unfamiliar with the means for obtaining drinking water. Arboreal lizards and snakes should be furnished with appropriate branches upon which to crawl or rest. Reptiles which are adapted to saline water must not be furnished with non-saline water, and vice versa. Those species that are best adapted to life in brackish water should be provided with diluted saline or artificial sea water that has been appropriately diluted to yield a half-strength concentration.

Fossorial (burrowing) species must be furnished with a suitable *nonresinous* substrate in which to burrow. Depending upon the requirements of each individual species, this substrate may be sandy loam, well-composted forest humus, leaf mold, or a similar material.

Secretive reptiles must be furnished with appropriate hiding places in which to seek refuge. Curved pieces of weathered oak bark, broken or inverted intact ceramic flowerpots, a length of ceramic drain pipe or roofing tile, or simply an inverted cardboard box with an entry hole can be employed for this purpose. Some highly active reptiles adapt poorly to the conditions of captivity and may "pace" the perimeters of their enclosures continually. The sexual dominance or territoriality of many species of reptiles, especially some lizards and chelonians, must be recognized and appropriate measures taken to lessen their negative effects. Overcrowding is a common shortcoming of many captive reptile environments and must be strictly avoided.

Because of their general heterothermia and need for the provision of external warmth for proper food digestion and assimilation, immune system function, and reproduction, an adequate and appropriate means for cage heating is essen-

GENERAL CONSIDERATIONS

tial. Undercage thermal heating pads, overhead radiant heating lights, heating stones, etc. have been used to good effect. The source of warmth must be tailored to match the thermal habits of each species. For instance, the use of heating blocks or stones usually is inappropriate for snakes and terrestrial chelonians because it is not their habit to coil or rest upon warm bodies—with the exception of some snakes that seek the warmth of black-top roads in the early evening hours. Placing an adjustable thermal heating pad beneath the cage will provide a steady and easily adjusted source of warmth without having an electrical cord left exposed in the cage. Overhead radiant heating lamps are used to form warm basking sites for species, especially diurnal lizards. When these lights are turned off so that an appropriate photoperiod is maintained, the under-cage heating pads or heat tapes help provide the necessary cage warmth. Large enclosures usually require multiple basking sites so that territorial disputes are lessened.

CHAPTER 2

NUTRITION

It is beyond the scope of this monograph to exhaust the intricacies of the various diets which must be fed to these fascinating animals; for those interested, see Frye (1991) **A PRACTICAL GUIDE FOR FEEDING CAPTIVE REPTILES**, Malabar, FL; Krieger Publ. Co. The following tables are reprinted (with minor additions and changes) from that text and will serve as a quick reference as to what the major species of reptile normally consume. Please note that most herbivorous and insectivorous reptiles should be fed diets which contain a calcium:phosphorus ratio of from approximately 1:1 to 2:1 in order to promote bone growth and maintenance.

When considering the health and welfare of any animal, the role of nutrition, with all of its gross and subtle ramifications, must be examined. Nutrition must be regarded as a continuum beginning with selection, apprehension or gathering of food sources, initial processing, digestion, assimilation of nutritive constituents and, finally, elimination of non-nutritive fibre, waste products, mucus, and senescent epithelial cells lining the alimentary tract. All of the bodily processes are linked in one way or another with nutrition. For instance, the immediate needs of the animal such as orderly growth and maintaining its cardiopulmonary, digestive, immune, hematopoietic, endocrine, reproductive, and nervous system functions are but a few of the vital processes that rely upon an adequate intake and processing of metabolites. Even the psychic "health" of a creature in captivity may, to a large part, be linked to the food that it is fed and the manner in which it is presented. Because moisture is intimately related to food processing, digestion, assimilation, fecal and urinary waste elimination, water consumption and its provision in a suitable manner must also be regarded. The condition of the food gathering organs often determines the ability of an individual to bite and/or chew its fare, swallow a bolus of food, and commence the initial and later processes of food digestion.

Because most reptiles are functionally hetero- or ectothermic, their deep-core body temperatures and, thus, their metabolism, are determined largely by external heat sources; therefore, the effects of inappropriate ambient temperature, as well as improper photoperiod and relative humidity, are often intimately associated with the overall nutrition and health of these animals.

Strictly speaking, there are few completely herbivorous or carnivorous reptiles—even obligatory herbivores consume plants that are often, if not almost always, infested with plant lice, mites, and other invertebrate animals. Consequently, some non-leguminous vegetables possess a high protein content (one need only examine flowerlet of fresh broccoli to prove this to be correct); therefore, most plant-eating or nectar-feeding prey also must be included in this category. When an obligate carnivore subdues and consumes an herbivorous prey animal, the carnivore swallows and benefits from the stomach and intestinal contents of its prey because these gut contents are rich in soluble vitamins and minerals.

A few predominantly herbivorous tortoises consume molluscs, carrion, and even the feces of other animals; valuable macro- and micronutrients are obtained from these sources. One of the few reptiles that truly subsists on a strictly animal protein diet is the egg-eating snake, *Dasypeltis scabra*; however, when eggs are not available, this snake may hunt for and eat rodents and birds and, therefore, consumes their gut contents. Sometimes, captive reptiles will develop the habit termed *pica* which is characterized by the purposeful ingestion of non-food items. One of the most common causes for this self-destructive behavior is boredom.

Most solitary or non-colonial animals usually display some degree of social dominance and territoriality, and the behavior of these creatures can determine success or failure when they are kept in captivity. Even when a splendid menu is offered to a group of reptiles, if one or more dominant individuals keep lower ranked creatures from a favored feeding site or a water source, the latter animals will fail to thrive and are likely to languish and die. Thus, the effects of interactive social stress and other forces on nutrition also must be considered. The deleterious consequences of human interference (conditioned by the very nature of captivity) can severely affect the appetite and, therefore, health of captive animals. Improper dietary supplementation with vitamins and minerals can lead directly or indirectly to iatrogenic or artificial diet-related vitamin or mineral imbalances and other nutritional disorders. The viewing public's nearly constant tapping on caged reptiles' terraria with a transparent front wall, and even the mere passage of people before such reptile cages, often are sufficiently distracting to induce anorexia because stressed animals are less likely to feed voluntarily.

Each of these topics will be discussed in this chapter in a "holistic" approach which considers the entire animal and the conditions of its captivity that may impinge upon its overall health—and survival.

PROVISION OF AN ADEQUATE WATER SUPPLY

Although some reptiles, particularly some highly specialized desert-dwellers, apparently do not require fluid water in their diet, most others must imbibe water at least occasionally. Some desert-inhabiting species of lizards such as the Australian moloch lizard, *Moloch horridus*, and many North American horned lizards, *Phrynosoma* sp., have, as a prime example of parallel evolution in two widely disparate but morphologically similar species, developed a system of interscalar channels through which water collected as dew on the spiny-scaled integument is conveyed into the corners of the animal's mouth by capillary action. (Sherbrooke, 1990).

Contrary to popular belief, reptiles do not absorb significant amounts of water through their skin. Many lizards imbibe water as rain- or dew-drops from foliage and often these species refuse to drink from vessels of standing water; others can be trained to accept water from one or more small emitters connected to a drip irrigation system. This watering scheme is useful when dealing with chameleons and arboreal iguanid lizards (Frye and Townsend, 1993). Some tree-dwelling snakes collect rain among their tightly held coils and, recently, this behavior has been recorded in a ground dwelling rattlesnake (Aird and Aird, 1990). Although many tortoises obtain a majority of their water from the moisture content of the succulent tissues of the various plants that they ingest, most, if not all, will drink eagerly if water is furnished in shallow pans or similar containers. The water must be sufficiently deep to permit the immersion of the external nares so that these animals can create a vacuum and, thus, draw the fluid into their mouths (they lack a shelf-like complete hard palate and the external nostrils must, therefore, be immersed beneath the water's surface). Relatively shallow bodies of water often may be available in the native habitat for only a very brief seasonally dictated time; the tortoises compensate for this by imbibing a large volume of water in a brief period of time; they further conserve vitally important amounts of water through osmotic reabsorption across the membrane of the urinary bladder. Many marine or pelagic reptiles are capable of imbibing sea water; the excess electrolytes are then secreted by specialized "salt glands" located in the nasal passages or beneath the tongue as a hyperosmolar product containing sodium, potassium, chloride, and minor amounts of trace minerals present in the saline water. Some terrestrial reptiles also possess similar salt-secreting glands from which they secrete concentrated electrolytes extra-renally without the loss of appreciable—and precious—water.

SELECTION OF FOOD

Some reptiles are highly selective in their choice of food; others are much less so. In some cases, there may be a selection of a particular type or class of food that contains a specific nutritional element that the reptile needs at that moment. Many wild-ranging terrestrial tortoises are attracted to carrion, dried skeletal remains, and even the feces of other animals. Many chelonians, particularly terrestrial tortoises, are able to discriminate bright colors; red, orange, yellow, and green are attractive to many, if not most, tortoises and some turtles. Motion is perceived acutely by many reptiles; thus, many chelonians, most lizards and snakes, crocodilians, and probably the tuatara, *Sphenodon punctatus*, are, to a large extent, sight-feeders. Few reptiles are attracted by auditory cues. Some reptiles possess one or more highly specialized nonvisual and nonauditory sense organs. The facial pit organs of the pit vipers and the labial pits of some boid snakes are examples of non-visual organs for the perception of both prey and potential predators. The vomeronasal (Jacobson's) organ is well developed in snakes and most lizards, and chemical or organoleptic cues are utilized extensively by these squamates and by some chelonians and most crocodilians. Fruit-eating skinks and geckos are attracted to sweet and nectar-rich fruits because of these lizards' ability to sense fragrant foods. Similarly, many tortoises are attracted to flavorful fruits and vegetables. Therefore, pleasant tasting nectars and pureés can be used as carrier media for vitamins and minerals which can be added to the diet to supplement important micronutrients. Some reptiles utilize extraoptical food detection techniques and can be attracted to food; often they can be induced to feed satisfactorily even when they lack their conventional sense of sight or their tongue as a result of a traumatic event or due to a developmental anomaly. Numerous reports describing anophthalmic reptiles and those affected by lingual aplasia have been recorded, and the author has observed several tongueless snakes and lizards and eyeless chelonians and snakes who have been trained to find and secure their food with minimal difficulty. These animals detect food by tactile or other stimuli furnished by their keepers.

A thorough knowledge of *which* animals prefer *what* specific dietary items is essential in order to provide a diet which is both attractive and accepted by captive reptiles and, at the same time, one which is nutritionally sound. It is useless to feed a fruit and/or leafy vegetable diet to an animal who will only dine upon fish, mice, or lizards. Moreover, the physical size, nutritional density, or quality and quantity of the preferred dietary items must be matched to the requirements of each individual reptile. For instance, very large boid snakes will find it nearly impossible to apprehend a small mouse; a very tiny kingsnake is far too small to apprehend, subdue, and swallow a large mouse, lizard, or snake. Placing surplus meal beetle larvae, crickets or other insects into a cage which houses lethargic lizards often results in the insects attacking and killing the reptiles in a quest for moisture and/or sustenance. Also, feeding in excess of what an animal can be reasonably expected to consume at one meal will result in obesity, food spoilage, promotion of fungal and/or bacterial growth, and attraction of insect vermin to the uneaten portions.

The quality of the diet is essential to the animal's health. Vegetables and fruit must be free from fungal infection, spoilage or other signs of decay. Dietary items that consist largely of indigestible non-nutritive fiber must be consumed in large quantity in order for them to yield sufficient digestible nutrients. Some plants have been associated with the induction of goiters and should not be fed excessively. These vegetables include cabbage and many of its relatives in the family

Brassicacae (Cruciferae): broccoli, Brussels sprouts, cauliflower, kale, kohlrabi, mustard, rutabagas, turnips, and others. Collard greens, a member of this richly diverse family, is much less likely to induce hypothyroidism and is highly nutritious and avidly eaten by many leaf-eating reptiles, particularly iguanas. Also, it possesses a calcium: phosphorus ratio that is well within the desired range (at least 2:1); that is, it contains much more calcium than phosphorus. Soy beans also contain goitrogenic substances. Generally, a *variety* of vegetables or other plant fodders should be fed; this will help avoid nutritional deficiencies and the development of undesirable habitual dietary preferences. It is relatively common for some reptiles to develop strong preferences for head lettuce, bananas, grapes, crickets, or mealworms and refuse to accept substitute and more nutritionally sound food items.

Animal prey should be free from pathology and, if possible, be tested periodically for the presence of bacterial infection and parasitic infestation. Fresh and frozen fish should be of highest quality to avoid fish-related diseases and nutritional disorders such as hypovitaminosis B_1 which is associated with the presence of the lytic enzyme thiaminase commonly present in improperly handled or stale fish and some shellfish. To avoid inducing steatitis, the inflammatory disorder which affects body fat, limit the feeding of fat-laden fish. Both disorders often can be avoided by feeding live fish to fish-eating reptiles.

In some instances, captive snakes prefer to attack and consume dark or naturally colored rodents and will refuse to attack or eat albino mice and rats. Egg-eating snakes readily accept freshly laid eggs gathered from the nest, but will reject cleaned eggs purchased from a grocery. Some large carrion-eating varanid lizards, crocodilians, and a few aquatic turtles may refuse to eat freshly killed food objects, preferring to wait until decomposition occurs (Auffenberg, 1981; Sprackland, 1990). It is now a common practice to warm quick-frozen rodents and fowl chicks in a microwave oven just before presenting them to some carnivorous reptiles, but it is essential to make certain that the internal temperature of these warmed items is not so hot that delicate oropharyngeal, esophageal, and gastric tissues are burned as the prey is swallowed. Crickets fed moldy poultry meal may contain sufficient aflatoxins to induce acute and chronic aflatoxicosis and, thus, severe liver disease, particularly toxic hepatitis in the insectivorous reptiles which eat them.

Some reptiles prefer unnatural diets that are nutritionally inadequate to meet their metabolic requirements for growth and maintenance. For instance, many tortoises and iguanine lizards avidly consume iceberg head lettuce, bananas, melons, cucumbers, tomatoes, and other plants which are deficient or poorly balanced in regard to essential minerals. Similarly, a diet restricted to meal beetle larvae or crickets often leads inexorably to metabolic bone disease. Vitamin-mineral supplementation must be employed when these nutritionally imperfect food items are fed, but great care must be exercised to avoid the vitamin overdosage and mineral imbalances that can be induced by such nutritional augmentation. To a large extent, the adage, "You are what you eat" applies to reptiles as well as to their human captors. Just as spoiled grapes are unlikely to yield a splendid vintage wine, decayed or otherwise poor quality foodstuffs are unlikely to

NUTRITION

support captive reptiles in a state of vigorous health. This requirement for high-quality fare is particularly germane when nursing care is given to traumatized reptiles; it is also important in the postoperative care of reptiles who are recovering from surgery.

Supplementing the captive diet with vitamins and mineral products can result in the induction of vitamin toxicities and imbalances between calcium, phosphorus and, to a lesser extent, magnesium and some trace minerals. Commercially prepared vitamins A and D are often provided in excessive amounts than are necessary for the normal growth and maintenance of reptiles. The vitamin A precursor, beta carotene, is usually well accepted and is substantially less toxic than the bioactive retinol (or retinyl ester), vitamin A; beta carotene can be furnished safely in the diet by feeding orange, yellow, and green leafy vegetables. Vitamin D, when fed excessively, can induce severe pathologic mineralization in normally non-calcified soft tissues such as smooth muscle that is present in the alimentary, respiratory, cardiovascular, and genitourinary organs. Moreover, an intimate interrelationship exists between *excessive* amounts of vitamin A and *deficient* amounts of vitamin D; it appears that excessive preformed vitamin A can initiate some of the physiologic and anatomic sequellae usually characteristic of vitamin D deficiency. Ingestion of excessive vitamin D and calcium also must be avoided. The precise mechanism of this competetive interrelationship is being studied at this time. The view has emerged that vitamin A should be supplied by feeding *natural* sources of beta carotene. Vitamin D should be furnished by the endogenous formation of this vitamin through the irradiation of cholesterol in the skin to 7-dehydrocholesterol, thence to Vitamin D_3 (cholecalciferol) to 25-hydroxycholecalciferol in the liver and, finally, to 1,25 dihydroxycholecalciferol in the kidneys; this cascade of metabolic events occurs when normal skin is exposed to either natural sunlight unfiltered through glass or to artificial ultraviolet lamps of sufficient chromatic index (90 or above) with or without additional "black" light augmentation.

APPREHENSION OF PREY AND GATHERING OF FODDER

Carnivorous or omnivorous reptiles pursue and apprehend their prey by simply grasping and immediately swallowing, aggressively attacking, envenomating, constricting, or other physical means of overpowering and restraining. Some employ more than one of these strategies, depending upon the amount of struggling by the prey animal. Even venomous reptiles may not envenomate a prey animal if it can be overcome by restraint alone. When prey is envenomated, it may or may not be released to die at some distance from the attacker. The venom used to subdue the prey may also play an important role in the enzymatic digestion of the meal. When a prey animal is too large to be swallowed whole, some lizards and most crocodilians twist their bodies while holding onto a piece of the animal, thus reducing the carcass to smaller portions that can be swallowed more easily.

Obligate herbivores and/or facultative omnivores grasp their vegetable food items with highly specialized toothless, yet often serrated, horn-covered nipping jaws, or with sharp-toothed mouths. Small pieces are snipped or avulsed from leafy vegetables; larger pieces are held down with a forelimb and then dismembered with the jaws into smaller bite-sized pieces before being swallowed—usually without mastication.

Some reptiles possess a highly cornified esophageal mucosa which resists abrasion by scabrous food items. Others are characterized by specialized structures which facilitate the ingestion of some food items. These structures include hard ridges in the roof of the esophagus such as those in the egg-eating snake, *Dasypeltus scabra*; as an egg passes under the ridges, powerful esophageal contractions compress the egg, slitting the shell and causing it to collapse and release its contents into the esophagus; the empty shell is then disgorged. Other reptiles, particularly many snakes, secrete copious amounts of slippery mucus with which their food is lubricated during swallowing. Some reptiles possess highly specialized teeth which reflect the nature of the diet. An example of this form of specialized dentition can be found in the caiman lizard, *Dracaena guianensis*: its diet consists of molluscs whose hard shells are crushed by the lizard's large, flat cusped molar-like teeth in order to extract the soft-bodied contents. Bird-eating snakes often possess long, recurved sharp teeth to better secure feathered prey; gharials, who dine largely upon fish, possess sharply pointed and elongated teeth which stud their narrow jaws. Other reptiles, especially some lizards, possess tongues whose tips have fine papillary projections and are liberally covered with sticky mucus; this arrangement facilitates capturing insects. Perhaps the most remarkable lingual adaptation is found in members of the lizard family Chameleonidae: the tongues of these lizards, when fully extended, often exceed the total length of the lizard. Lying in the floor of the mouth when not deployed, these astonishing organs can be extended and withdrawn very rapidly, thus capturing and retrieving ordinarily wary flying insects. Some leaf-eating lizards possess a partially compartmentalized large bowel that serves a fermentation vessel during hindgut processing of cellulose by microorganisms. Many of the iguanine lizards also employ this form of hindgut digestion.

Because many reptiles are quiescent in captivity, their expenditure of energy in foraging for food or other energy-expending activities are greatly diminished compared to the same animals who are wild and have to hunt for their livelihood. Consequently, overfeeding and obesity are commonly observed in many of the less active species. Some captive reptiles, because of their high activity level, must be fed often just to maintain their normal weight. The nature of the diet is extremely important when ascertaining the frequency of feeding: items high in water content and low in dry matter, or high in fibre, contain less utilizable energy when compared to more concentrated items which contain less moisture or fiber, or are rich in fats.

Boredom often accompanies captivity. Many reptiles do little in captivity other than eat, drink, eliminate wastes, slough their senescent skin and, occasionally, mate. The majority of their time is spent in enforced idleness. In many instances, these animals appear physically to be unaffected; in other cases, most of the reptile's time is consumed in attempts to escape or in inappropriate repetitive "pacing" behaviors that often result in self-induced trauma from constant abrasion of the animal's rostrum against the cage walls or other unyielding surfaces. In some cases, captive reptiles will develop the habit of ingesting cage litter materials. This consumption of indigestible particulate material such as sand, pebbles, wood chips, ground corn (maize) cobs, sawdust, moss, cat litter, etc., can lead inexorably to gastrointestinal obstruction and eventual death.

Sometimes, this excessive "free" time can be channeled into more constructive activities such as prey pursuit. If live fish are placed in a container of water, the predator reptile must spend much more energy (and surplus time) in foraging and capturing prey rather than merely being fed pre-killed, thawed frozen fish; this more closely approximates the situation present under natural conditions. The diet of obese, sedentary herbivorous reptiles should be changed to include more high-fiber vegetation and high-water content succulent fruit and less bread, starches, or sugar-laden ripe fruit or other energy-rich items.

INITIAL PROCESSING

Depending upon the nature of the individual reptile under consideration, the meal may be swallowed whole (as by snakes, some lizards, some chelonians, and some crocodilians) or chewed before it is devoured. Those animals who ingest the entire meal as intact prey are less likely to develop nutritional deficiency disorders because not only are the soft tissues of the prey ingested, but the entire mineral-rich skeleton, plus fur, feathers, or scales and, importantly, the stomach contents that were eaten by the prey prior to it being swallowed by the predator also are ingested.

In some instances, the venom that helped subdue the prey may also initiate the early stages of the digestive process. In snakes which lack a venom or venom-delivery apparatus due to prior surgical intervention, the digestive process may be impeded by the absence of venom which is often enzyme-rich and aids in the initial digestion of the prey (Klauber, 1956). The act of striking and biting often serves as a powerful releaser for feeding behavior in snakes. Similarly, the hunting and attack sequences characteristic of many crocodilians' feeding behavior serve as stimuli to feeding and swallowing. It is for this reason that when many crocodilians are housed under crowded conditions, they may exhibit "feeding frenzies" during which their cohorts are injured. To a lesser extent, these frenzied episodes can occur in turtles and some carnivorous lizards, especially large varanids.

In those instances where active mastication precedes engulfing, the meal is triturated, mixed with saliva, and finally swallowed. Thus, by the time the food enters the stomach, it is partially macerated and may be reduced in particle size, therefore increasing the surface area upon which the enzyme-rich digestive secretions can act. In some cases, animals will purposely ingest stones which aid in the maceration process. These stones often serve another function as well: they aid in maintaining negative buoyancy by adding mass to the animal. Fresh water aquatic turtles and crocodilians employ this technique in order to remain submerged. When these animals are kept in captivity, particularly under conditions of public display, this stone eating behavior (*lithophagy*) may be replaced by the potentially harmful ingestion of man-made foreign bodies such as coins and tokens, bottle caps, nursing nipples, cosmetic jewelry, toys, etc; this must be prevented.

Most snakes, crocodilians, carnivorous lizards and chelonians, and the tuatara possess gland-rich gastric mucosae that rapidly digest the complex animal prey meals that these creatures ingest. The bone-rich meals become demineralized and digested within three or four days of being swallowed. Even the teeth of some prey are softened by these potent acidic gastric secretions.

ASSIMILATION

Ingested food is partially digested in the stomach, thence moves into the small intestine where it is mixed with pancreatic enzyme-rich digestive secretions and bile and is further digested. This sequence of events depends upon the size and nature of the meal, ambient temperature, physical condition of the animal, and the presence or absence of gastrointestinal parasitism. Eventually, protein-, fat- and, to a variable extent, carbohydrate-laden nutrients are absorbed into the bloodstream. The blood flowing from the intestines travels first to the liver where the basic "building blocks" consisting of amino acids and peptides, fatty acids, di- and triglycerides, lipoproteins, and mono-, di-, oligo- and polysaccharides are extracted, stored, and processed into other bioactive products. It is from these molecules that the protein, fat, cellulose, starches and plant gums in the diet are formed. In addition, essential vitamins, enzymes, trace minerals and co-factors are absorbed and converted to substances from which body tissues are formed and maintained.

Enzymatic degradation that is responsible for digestion of proteins, fats, and carbohydrates is largely temperature-dependent: at temperatures lower than their optimal (Michaelis) constant, the activity of each enzyme is diminished; conversely, raising the temperature tends to increase each enzyme's activity up to a maximum which differs with each individual enzyme. Beyond this point, further temperature elevation results in reduced catalytic activity.

Many reptiles become quiescent after ingesting a large meal. Some snakes and large monitor lizards may remain inactive for many days while the digestive process continues. Under natural conditions, the postprandial act of moving to a safe refuge in which to hide may stimulate digestion and help reduce intestinal gas production by increasing peristaltic motility, and the ambient temperatures tend to fluctuate between maximum and minimum during a 24-hour cycle. Under captive conditions, however, exercise is limited because of cage space constraints, and the ambient temperature tends to remain at a relatively constant level; most often, this temperature is close to the preferred optimum for a particular species. Unfortunately, the lack of exercise and the level warm temperature favor the production—and retention—of intestinal gas. Because many long-term captive giant snakes are already obese, this form of captive habitat-related flatulence is exacerbated and can become life-threatening if not treated vigorously with encouraged exercise and gas-lysing agents such as simethicone given by stomach тube. Permitting and encouraging the affected reptile (usually a giant boid snake) to swim, facilitates the lysis and/or passage of this gas as flatus. Once remedial action is taken, relief of this condition can be dramatic.

ELIMINATION

Mammal-eating and bird-eating reptiles tend to have bulky fur- or feather-laden feces. Since many of these animals, under wild conditions, vary their diet between several kinds of prey, fur and feather impactions are probably rare occurrences. However, under captive conditions when the diet is not varied, these impactions are commonly encountered and must be treated with stool softeners and lubricative laxative products. Impactions can be avoided by feeding mammal and bird prey alternately.

Herbivorous reptiles, because of their high fiber diet, tend to require a relatively long transit time between ingestion and defecation, and their feces tend to be more bulky and more frequently passed than those of a carnivorous reptile. When fed a succulent diet with a very high water intake such as squashes, melons, and cucumbers, the feces of many tortoises tend to be near-liquid in consistency. Microscopic examination for parasites should be part of the evaluation of any case of diarrhea, but if the analysis is negative for pathogens, frank diarrhea can often be treated effectively by changing the diet to a much drier fiber-rich ration. One remedy that has proven very effective in firming previously loose stools is the feeding of pelleted alfalfa hay. The pellet size ranges from the smallest fed to rabbits and other diminutive herbivorous mammals to the large compressed flakes fed to large hoofed stock; the size should be matched to the animals to whom it is fed.

Some cage litter materials can be accidentally ingested along with the meal and, if not regurgitated, can cause gastrointestinal obstruction or mucosal inflammation. Examples of these substances are ground corncob, some forms of wood shavings or wood wool, cat litter, sand, small pebbles, etc. Their most benign effect is to cause discomfort. More serious effects are mucosal erosion; ulceration; perforation of the stomach or intestines; partial lumenal obstruction; intussusception; or complete obstruction which prevents passage of ingesta and/or feces.

MISCELLANEOUS FACTORS AND THEIR EFFECTS ON NUTRITION

As noted earlier, stress that impinges upon nutrition and health can arise from any of several conditions common to captivity. The importance of avoiding stress cannot be overemphasized. Examples of the major causes for stress are: thirst; hunger; improper diet; inadequate or excessive environmental temperature, humidity, or photoperiod; overcrowding; poorly matched social dominance or sexually established territoriality; physical or metabolic disturbances; psychic stress from human:reptile interactions; housing which lacks appropriate hiding refuges; housing prey species with their potential predators; differences in the size of cagemates; the presence of infectious or parasitic disease; during recovery from infectious, parasitic, or metabolic disease; during the postoperative period of healing following surgery; courtship including male-to-male combat; and the production of sperm, eggs, or embryos. Each of these stressors can result in a lack of/or diminished appetite; when more than one is present, the effect can be devastating, particularly in chameleons, some iguanids, agamids and other usually solitary lizards.

TABLE 1
FOOD PREFERENCES FOR SELECTED SNAKE SPECIES

SNAKE	SM	B	OS	L	E	F/T/S	F	I/A	W/S
AESCULAPIAN SNAKE *Elaphe l. longissimus*	X	O							
AFRICAN BEAKED SNAKE *Rhamphiophis multimaculatus*	X			O					
AFRICAN HOUSE SNAKE *Lamprophis fulginosus*	X	X		O	O				
ANACONDA *Eunectes murinus,* *Eunectes notaeus*	X	X	X	O	O	O	X	O	
ARGENTINE GREEN SPECKLED SNAKE *Leimadophis poecilogyrus*							small live fish		
ASIAN RAT SNAKE (MANGROVE RAT SNAKE) *Gonyosoma* sp.	X	X							
AUSTRALIAN TREE SNAKE *Dendrelaphis punctularus*	X	X		O		X			

30

Snake							
BANDY-BANDY SNAKE *Vermicella annulata*			X				
BIRD SNAKE *Thelotornis kirtlandii*	X	X	X	X			
BLACK-HEADED *Tantilla* sp.						X	O insect larvae and arachnids
BLACK-STRIPED *Coniophanes imperialis*	X	X	X	X			
BLACK SWAMP SNAKE *Seminatrix* sp.					O	X	earthworms
BLIND *Rhamphotyphlops* etc.			O			X	
BLUNT-HEADED TREE SNAKE *Imantodes cenchoa*			X				
BOA/PYTHON *Aspidites, Boa, Calabaria, Candoia, Charina, Chondropython, Corallus, Exiliboa, Epicrates, Eryx, Liasis, Lichanura, Morelia, Python, Trachyboa, Tropidophis, Ungaliophis,* etc.	X	X	X	O	O	O in some dwarf boas	
BOOMSLANG *Dispholidus typus*	X	X	X	O	O		

31

SNAKE	SM	B	OS	L	E	F/T/S	F	I/A	W/S
BROWN TREE *Boiga irregularis*	X	X			X	O		O	
BULL SNAKE *Pituophis melanoleucus*	X	X							
BUSHMASTER *Lachesis muta muta*	X	X				frogs			
CANTIL *Agkistrodon bilineatus*	X	O	X	O		X	X		
CAT-EYED, NORTH AMERICAN *Leptodeira septentrionalis*;				X		X			
CAT-EYED, SOUTH AMERICAN *Boiga* sp.	X	X		X					
COACHWHIP *Masticophis* sp.	X	X	O	X	O	O		O	
COBRA (Exc. King Cobra) *Aspidelaps* sp.; *Boulengerina* sp.; *Hemachatus haemachatus*; *Naja* sp., *Pseudohaje goldii*; *Walterinnesia aegyptiae*	X quail chicks	X	O	O					
COPPERHEAD *Agkistrodon contortrix*	X	O	O	O	O	X	O	cicadas & larvae	

COPPERHEAD RACER *Elaphe radiata*	X	X			
CORAL *Micrurus* sp. *Micruroides* sp.	mouse pups		X	X	O
CORN SNAKE *Elaphe guttata*	X	X			
CRAWFISH or SWAMP *Regina* sp.				amphibians X & their larvae	crawfish & aquatic nymphs
CRIBO *Drymarchon corais*	X	X	X	X	
CROWNED SNAKE, NEW WORLD *Tantilla* sp.		X	X		X
CROWNED SNAKE, OLD WORLD *Coronella girondica*	X	X	X		X as juveniles
DEATH ADDER *Acanthophis antarticus*	X	X	X		
DeKAY'S *Storeria dekayi*				X tiny salamanders	X
DIADEM SNAKE *Spalerosophis diadema*	X	X	X		

SNAKE	SM	B	OS	L	E	F/T/S	F	I/A	W/S
EARTH SNAKE (ROUGH): *Virginia striatula* (SMOOTH): *Virginia valeriae*						X		X	X
EGG-EATING *Dasypeltis scabra*	O	O			X				
ELEPHANT TRUNK or KARUNG *Acrochordus sp.*							X goldfish		
FALSE CORAL SNAKE *Anilius scytale*			X	X		X			
FALSE CORAL SNAKE *Erythrolampus bizona*	X		X	X					
FALSE HABU *Macropisthodon rudis*			X	X		X			
FALSE WATER COBRA; BRAZILIAN SMOOTH SNAKE *Cyclagras gigas*			X			X	X		
FLAT-HEADED SNAKE *Tantilla gracilis*								X	X
FOX SNAKE *Elaphe vulpina*	X	X							

GARTER, RIBBON *Thamnophis* sp.	X	X	O	X	O		X	X	X
GLOSSY SNAKE *Arizona elegans*	X		X	X				O	
GOPHER, BULL, PINE *Pituophis melanoleucus* spp.	X	X			O				
GREEN *Opheodrys* sp. *Liopeltis* sp.		O	O	X	X	O		X	O
GROUND SNAKE *Sonora semiannulata*								X	
HERALD SNAKE *Crotaphopeltis botamboeia*					X	O			
HOG-NOSED *Heterodon* sp.; *Leioheterodon madagascariensis*; *Xenodon* sp.	O		O rarely	O	X	O			
HOOK-NOSED *Glyalopion* sp. *Ficimia streckeri*								X	
INDIGO *Drymarchon* sp.	X	X	X	X	X			O	O

SNAKE	SM	B	OS	L	E	F/T/S	F	I/A	W/S
KEELED RAT SNAKE *Zaocys dhumnades*	X	X	O	O		X			
KINGSNAKE *Lampropeltis* sp.	X	X	X	X	O	O		O	
KING COBRA *Ophiophagus*	O		X	X					
KIRTLAND'S *Clonophis kirtlandi*									X
KRAIT *Bungarus* sp.	X			X	X	O			
LEAF-NOSED *Phyllorhynchus decurtatus*				X					
LINED *Tropidoclonium lineatum*						X	X	O	
LONG-NOSED *Rhinocheilus lecontei*	X		X and their eggs	X					
LYRE *Trimorphodon biscutatus*	X	X	X	X					X

MALAYAN LONG-GLANDED CORAL SNAKE *Maticora bivirgata flaviceps*			x	x
MAMBA *Dendraspis* sp.	x	x	o	x
MANGROVE *Boiga dendrophila*	x	x		x	o
MARINE/SEA *Acalyptophis peronii*; *Aipysurus* sp.; *Astrotia stokesii*; *Emydocephalus* sp. *Hydrophis*; *Laticauda* sp. *Lapemis* sp.; *Pelamis platurus*					x
MILK SNAKE *Lampropeltis triangulum*	x	x	x	x
MOHAGANY RAT SNAKE "PUFFING" SNAKE *Pseutes* sp.	x	x		x	o as juveniles
MOLE SNAKE *Lampropeltis calligaster rhombomaculata*; *Pseudaspis cana*	x	x		x

SNAKE	SM	B	OS	L	E	F/T/S	F	I/A	W/S
MONPELLIER SNAKE *Malpolon* sp.	X	X							
MUD *Farancia abacura*					salamanders esp. *Amphiuma*				
MUSSURANA *Clelia clelia*	X		X	O					
NECK-BANDED *Scaphiodontophis annulatus bondurensis*				X					
NIGHT/CAT-EYED *Eridiphas* sp., *Hypsiglena* sp., etc.	X	X	X	X		O		O	
PARROT SNAKE *Leptophis ahaetulla* *Chrysolopea* sp.				X		X			
PATCH-NOSED SNAKE *Salvadora* sp.				X and lizard eggs					
PINE SNAKE *Pituophis melanoleucus*	X	X							
PIPE SNAKE *Cylindrophis rufus*	X		X						

PIT VIPERS, ASIAN *Agkistrodon* sp.; *Calloselasma* sp.; *Deinagkistrodon acutus*; *Trimeresurus* sp.	×	O		×	O
PIT VIPERS, NEW WORLD *Agkistrodon* sp.; *Bothrops* sp.; *Bothriechis* sp.; *Crotalus* sp.; *Lachesis muta*; *Ophryacus* sp.; *Porthidium* sp.; *Sistrurus*, sp.	×	O		×	O O in some species
PYGMY RATTLESNAKE *Sistrurus miliarius*	×	O		×	
QUEEN SNAKE *Regina septemvittata*					crayfish
RACER (NEW WORLD) *Alsophis* sp.; *Coluber* sp.; *Drymobius* sp.; *Drymoluber* sp.	×	×	×	×	O O
RACER (OLD WORLD) *Haemorrhois* sp.; *Chironius* sp.	×	×		O	O
RAINBOW *Farancia erythrogramma*				tadpoles	

SNAKE	SM	B	OS	L	E	F/T/S	F	I/A	W/S
RAT/CHICKEN *Elaphe* sp.	X	X			X				
RATTLESNAKE *Crotalus* sp. *Sistrurus* sp.	X	X	X	X		O esp. the Massasauga		O	
RED-BELLIED *Storeria occipitomaculata*								X	X
RED-NECKED KEELBACK *Rhabdophis subminiatus*						X	X		
RIBBON *Thamnophis* sp.	X	O	X	X	X	X	O		X
RINGED SNAKE, GRASS SNAKE *Natrix natrix*						X	X		
RING-NECKED *Diadophis* sp.			O	O		X		O	X
SAND SNAKE *Psammophis* sp.	O			X				X	
SCARLET SNAKE *Cemophora coccinea*	X	X		X	X				
SHARP-TAILED *Contia tenuis*									slugs

SHORT-TAILED *Stilosoma extenuatum*		X	X		
SHOVEL-NOSED *Chionactes* sp.				X	
SNAIL-EATING *Dipsas indica; Sibon;* *Tropidodipsas sartori*					snails & slugs
SPECKLED SNAKE *Leimadophis* sp.	O	O	X	X	
SUNBEAM SNAKE *Xenopeltis unicolor*	X	X	X		
TAIPAN SNAKE *Oxyuranus scutellatus*	X				
TENTACLED SNAKE *Erpeton tentaculum*					small live fish
TIGER SNAKE *Notechis scutatus*	X	X	X		
TROPICAL CHICKEN *Spilotes pullatus*	X	X	X		
VINE SNAKES *Ahaetulla* sp.; *Oxybelis* sp. *Uromacer* sp.	O	X			

SNAKE	SM	B	OS	L	E	F/T/S	F	I/A	W/S
VIPERS, MISC.	X	X	O	X		O	O	O	O
Agkistrodon sp.; *Atheris* sp.;								esp. as	
Azemiops feae; *Bitis* sp.;								neonates	
Bothriechis sp.; *Bothrops* sp.;									
Calloselasma sp.; *Causus* sp.;									
Cerastes sp.; *Deinagkistrodon* sp.;									
Echis sp.; *Eristocophis* sp.;									
Lachesis muta; *Porthidium* sp.;									
Trimeresurus sp.; *Vipera* sp.									
WATER MOCCASIN	X	X	O	X		X	X	O	O
Agkistrodon piscivorus								esp. as	
								neonates	
WATERSNAKES	O		O			X	X	O	O
Nerodia sp.;								esp. as	
Natrix sp.								neonates	
WHIP SNAKE	X	X		X					
Masticophis sp.									

42

WOLF SNAKE *Lycodon* sp.; *Lycophidion* sp.	O	X	X	
WORM SNAKES *Typhlops* sp.; *Leptotyphlops*			X	termites, worms & grubs
YELLOW-LIPPED or PINE WOODS *Rhadinaea flavilata*		X	X	

LEGEND:
- X = usual food items
- B = birds
- E = eggs (avian & reptilian)
- F = fish
- W/S = worms, slugs & snails
- O = occasionally eaten
- OS = other snakes
- F/T/S = frogs, toads, salamanders
- SM = small mammals
- L = lizards
- I/A = insects & arachnids

TABLE 2
FOOD PREFERENCES FOR SELECTED LIZARD SPECIES

LIZARD SPECIES	SM	B	I	E	CM	M/G	FISH	FR/V
AGAMA *Agama* sp.	X		X and arachnids					O
ALLIGATOR *Elgaria* sp.	X	X	X and arachnids	O	X	O		
AMERICAN ANOLE *Anolis* sp.			X and arachnids					
ARMADILLO *Cordylus* sp.			X					O fruit
BASILISK *Basiliscus* sp.	X quail chicks		X and arachnids					O
BEADED, MEXICAN *Heloderma horridum*	X	X	O	X	X	O		O
BEARDED *Amphibolurus barbatus* *Pogona* sp.	X	O	X and arachnids	O	O	O	X	X
BRAZILIAN TREE LIZARD *Enhyalius catenatus*			X and arachnids					

CAIMAN *Dracaena guianensis*				clams/snails	X
CHAMELEON OLD WORLD *Chamaeleo* sp.	O#	X and arachnids		snails	O
CHUCKWALLA *Sauromalus* sp.	O	O	O		X
			boiled		
COLLARED *Crotaphytus* sp.	X	O	X and arachnids	O	X blossoms
CURLY-TAILED *Leiocephalus carinatus*			X and arachnids		
DEAF AGAMIDS *Cophotis* sp.			X and arachnids		
DWARF SAND LIZARD *Eremias grammica*			X and arachnids		
EARLESS *Holbrookia* sp., *Cophosaurus texanus*			X and arachnids		
FLYING DRAGON *Draco volans*			X and arachnids		
FRILLED LIZARD *Chlamydosaurus kingii*			X and arachnids		

LIZARD SPECIES	SM	B	I	E	CM	M/G	FISH	FR/V
FRINGE-TOED *Uma* sp.			X and arachnids					
GECKO, MISC. *Gekko, Hemidactylus, Coleonyx,* *Gehyra, Gonatodes, Hemitheconyx* *Phelsuma, Chondrodactylus,* *Nephrurus, Phyllodactylus* *Ptyodactylus, Tarentola,* *Sphaerodactylus* sp., etc.	X	O	X and arachnids	O				X fruit puree
GILA "MONSTER" *Heloderma suspectum*	X	X	O	X	X	O		O
GIRDLED LIZARD *Zonosaurus* sp.			X					O
GLASS LIZARD "SHELTOPUSIK" *Ophisaurus ventralis*	X	X	X	O	X	snails		
HELMETED LIZARD *Corythophanes* sp.			X and arachnids					
HORNED LIZARD *Phrynosoma* sp.			ants termites					

46

IGUANA, COMMON* *Iguana iguana;* *Iguana i. rhinolopha* *diet varies with age; see text	O	O	X	X	O	O	X esp. leafy
IGUANA, DESERT *Dipsosaurus dorsalis*	O		X	O	O		X
IGUANA, FIJI *Brachylophus* sp.	O	O	O	O	O		X
IGUANA, GROUND *Cyclura* sp., *Conolophus pallidus,*	X	O	O	O	O	X	X
IGUANA, MARINE *Amblyrhynchus* sp.					O	X	algae kelp
JUNGLE RUNNER *Ameiva ameiva*		X also arachnids & other lizards					
LACERTA, MISC. *Lacerta* sp.; *Gallotia stelini*	X	quail chicks	X	O	O		O
LEGLESS *Anniella pulcra*		X and arachnids					
LEOPARD *Gambelia* sp.		X also arachnids & other lizards					

LIZARD SPECIES	SM	B	I	E	CM	M/G	FISH	FR/V
LONG-TAILED BRUSH *Urosaurus graciosus*			X and arachnids					
LYRE-HEADED LIZARD *Lyriocephalus scutatus*			X and arachnids					
MOLOCH *Moloch horridus*			ants & termites					
MONITOR(S), MISC. *Varanus sp.* (except Gray's,	X	X	O	X	carrion		O	
GRAY'S MONITOR *V. olivaceus (V. grayi)*	O	O	O	O	O	X snails		X figs
MOUNTAIN LIZARD *Japalura sp.*			ants & termites					
MOUTAIN HORNED LIZARD *Acanthosaurus armata*			X and arachnids					
NIGHT *Xantusia sp.;* *Cricosaura typica*			ants & termites					

PLATED *Gerrhosaurus* sp.	X	X and arachnids	X	O	O
ROCK, BANDED *Petrosaurus mearnsi*		X and arachnids			
RUIN *Podarcis sicula*				O	X
RUSSIAN GARGOYLE LIZARD *Phrynocephalus mystaceus*		X and arachnids			
SAIL-TAILED *Hydrosaurus amboinensis*	X	O	O	X	X fruits, leaves & seeds
SAND LIZARDS *Psammodromus* sp.		X and arachnids			
SHARP-SNOUTED SNAKE LIZARD *Lialis burtonis*	other lizards	X			
SHELTOPUSIK *Ophisaurus apodus*	X	X	X	X	
SIDE-BLOTCHED *Uta stansburiana*		X and arachnids			

LIZARD SPECIES	SM	B	I	E	CM	M/G	FISH	FR/V
SKINK, MISC. (Old World & Australasian) *Scincus, Tiliqua, Chalcides, Trachydosaurus, Corucia zebrata*	O	O	O	O	O	O	O	X fruit puree & nectar
SKINKS, SMALL *Eumeces, Sincella, Neoceps reynoldsi; Lerista* sp.			X small arthropods & arachnids			snails		
SLOW "WORM" *Anguis fragilis*	O		X	O	X	O		
SNAKE LIZARD *Delma fraseri; Chamaesaura anguina*			X and arachnids					
SPINY *Sceloporus* sp.	X		X and arachnids					
SPINY-TAILED *Uromastix* sp.	X	O quail chicks	X	O	O			leafy plants, blossoms, & fruit
SPINY-TAILED IGUANAS *Ctenosaura pectinata; Urocentron* sp.			O			O		leafy plants, blossoms, & fruit

SUNGAZER LIZARD *Cordylus* sp.		X			X
SWIFT, FENCE, PLATEAU, SCRUB, ROSE-BELLIED, BUNCH GRASS, MESQUITE, SAGEBRUSH, etc. *Sceloporus* sp.	X	X and arachnids			
SWIFTS, SOUTH AMERICAN *Liolaemus* sp.		X and arachnids			
TEGU *Tupinambis* sp.	X	X and arachnids	X	X	X
THORNY DEVIL LIZARD *Heteropterex dilatata*		X and arachnids			
TREE or BRUSH LIZARDS *Urosaurus* sp.		X and arachnids			
WATER "DRAGON" *Physignathus leseurii*; *P. concincinus*	O	O	X fish	X snails	O
WHIP-TAILED *Cnemidophorus* sp.	O	X and arachnids		O	
WORM *Bipes biporus*, *Blanus*, *Rhineura floridana*		termites & tiny grubs		X live fish earthworms	

LIZARD SPECIES	SM	B	I	E	CM	M/G	FISH	FR/V
ZEBRA-TAILED *Callisaurus draconoides*			X and arachnids					

#esp. *C. parsoni* and *C. calyptratus*
LEGEND: X = usual food
B = birds
CM = chopped meats*
O = occasionally eaten
I = insects & arachnids
M/G = molluscs and gastropods
FR/V = fruits/vegetables*
SM = small mammals
E = eggs (avian & reptilian)

*may be supplemented with calcium carbonate (see text)

TABLE 3
FOOD PREFERENCES FOR SELECTED TURTLES, TERRAPINS, AND TORTOISES

CHELONIAN SPECIES	M	F	I/W/S/DF	FL	FR	V
AFRICAN HELMETED TURTLE *Pelomedusa subrufa*	X	X	X			pond weeds & algae
AFRICAN SIDE-NECKED TURTLES *Pelusios* sp.	X	X	X			pond weeds & algae
ALDABRA TORTOISE *Geochelone (Testudo) gigantea (Aldabrachelys elephantina*)*	O		O	X	X	X
ALLIGATOR SNAPPING TURTLE *Macrochelys temminckii*	X	X	X			
ARGENTINE SIDE-NECKED TURTLES *Phrynops* sp., *Hydromedusa tectifera*	X	X	crayfish			pond weeds & algae
ASIAN BOX TURTLES *Cuora* sp.	O	X	X	O	O	O
BIG-HEADED TURTLE *Platemys macrocephala*	X	X	X			pond weeds & algae

CHELONIAN SPECIES	M	F	I/W/S/DF	FL	FR	V
BLACK POND TURTLE *Seibenrockiella crassicollis*	X	X	X			pond weeds & algae
BLANDING'S TURTLE *Emydoidea blandingi*	X (juveniles tend to be more carnivorous than adults)	X	X	O		pond weeds & algae
BOG TURTLE *Clemmys muhlenbergi*	X	X	X			O
BOLSON TORTOISE *Gopherus (Xerobates) flavomarginata*			O	X	X	X
BOX TURTLE *Terrepene* sp.	X	O	X	X	X	X
BRAHMINY RIVER TURTLE *Hardella thurgi*	X	X	X			pond weeds & algae
BRAZILIAN SNAKE-NECKED *Hydromedusa maximiliani*	X	X	crayfish			pond weeds & algae
BURMESE MOUNTAIN TORTOISE *Geochelone emys*			snails	X	X	X
CHACO TORTOISE *Chelonoidis chilensis*	O		O	X	X	X

Species					
CHICKEN TURTLE *Deirochelys reticularia*	X	X		O	pond weeds & algae
	(juveniles tend to be more carnivorous than adults)				
COOTER *Chrysemys sp.*	X	X			pond weeds & algae
	(juveniles tend to be more carnivorous than adults)				
DESERT TORTOISE *Gopherus (Xerobates) agassizi*	O	O		X	X
		small amts DF			
DIAMONDBACK TERRAPIN *Malaclemys terrapin*	O	X	X esp. marine snails (periwinkles) small crabs		pond weeds & algae
EGYPTIAN TORTOISE *Testudo kleinmanni*		O		X	X
ELONGATED TORTOISE *Geochelone elongata*		X		X	X
FALSE MAP TURTLE *Graptemys pseudogeographica*	X	X		X	pond weeds & algae
FLY RIVER TURTLE *Carettochelys insculpta*	X	X		X	pond weeds & algae

CHELONIAN SPECIES	M	F	I/W/S/DF	FL	FR	V
FOUR-EYED TURTLE *Sacalia bealei*	O	X	X			pond weeds & algae
GALAPAGOS TORTOISE *Geochelone elephantopus* sp.	O		X	X	X	X
GOPHER TORTOISE *Gopherus polyphemus*	O		O	X	X	X
GREEK TORTOISE *Testudo graeca*	O		O	X	X	X
GREEN TURTLE, MARINE *Chelonia mydas* JUVENILES ADULTS	molluscs, crabs, & sponges	O	X			kelp algae
HAWKSBILL TURTLE *Eretmochelys imbricata* JUVENILES ADULTS	molluscs, crabs, & sponges	O				kelp algae
HERMANN'S TORTOISE *Testudo hermanni*	O		X	X	X	X
HINGEBACK TORTOISE *Kinexys* sp.	O		X	X	X	X

Species						
IMPRESSED TORTOISE *Geochelone impressa*	O		X	X	X	X
LEAF TURTLES, ASIAN *Cyclemys* sp.	X		X earthworms			X algae
LEATHERBACK TURTLE *Dermochelys coriacea* JUVENILES: ADULTS:	jellyfish jellyfish crabs, sponges & corals	X O				kelp algae
LEOPARD TORTOISE *Geochelone pardalis*	O	O	O	X	X	X
LOGGERHEAD TURTLE *Carretta carretta*	sponges crabs, & coral	O				O seaweed
LONG-NECKED *Chelodina longicollis*	O	X	X			
MAP TURTLE *Graptemys* sp.	X (juveniles tend to be more carnivorous than adults)	X	X			pond weeds & algae
MATA MATA TURTLE *Chelys fimbriata*	O	X	O			
MUD TURTLE *Kinosternon* sp.	X	X live	X			pond weeds & algae

57

CHELONIAN SPECIES	M	F	I/W/S/DF	FL	FR	V
MUHLENBERG'S TURTLE *Clemmys muhlenbergi*	X	X (juveniles tend to be more carnivorous than adults)				pond weeds & algae
MUSK TURTLE *Sternotherus* sp.	X	X	X			pond weeds & algae
NEW GUINEA SIDE-NECK TURTLE *Elysea novaguineae*	O	X	X			pond weeds & algae
OLIVE RIDLEY *Lepidochelys olivacea*		X	molluscs crabs, sponges, & corals			
PAINTED TURTLE *Chrysemys picta*	X	X (juveniles tend to be more carnivorous than adults)	X			pond weeds & algae
PANCAKE TORTOISE *Malachocherus tornieri* *M. procteri*			X	X	X	X
POND TURTLE *Clemmys* sp.	X	X (juveniles tend to be more carnivorous than adults)	X			pond weeds & algae

RADIATED TORTOISE *Geochelone radiata*	O	O		X	X
RED-EARED SLIDER TURT. *Trachemys** scripta elegans*	X	X (juveniles tend to be more carnivorous than adults)			pond weeds & algae
RED-FOOTED TORTOISE *Geochelone carbonaria*	O	X		X	X
REEVE'S TURTLE *Chinemys reevesi*	X	X			pond weeds & algae
RINGED SAWBACK TURTLE *Graptemys oculifera*	X	X			pond weeds & algae
SIDE-NECKED TURTLE *Chelodina sp.*, etc.	X	X			pond weeds & algae
SNAPPING TURTLE, COM. *Chelydra serpentina*	X	X			
SOFT-SHELLED *Apalone sp., Trionyx sp.*, etc.	X	X			
SOUTH AMERICAN RIVER TURTLE *Dermatemys mawei*	X	X			pond weeds & algae
SPOTTED TURTLE *Clemmys guttata*	X	X			pond weeds & algae

CHELONIAN SPECIES	M	F	I/W/S/DF	FL	FR	V
SPUR-THIGHED TORTOISE *Geochelone sulcata*			O	X	X	X
STAR TORTOISE *Geochelone elegans*	O		X	X	X	X
TOAD-HEADED *Phrynops* sp.		X	X			pond weeds & algae
WOOD TURTLE *Clemmys insculpta*	X	O	X		O	O
YELLOW-FOOTED TORT. *Geochelone denticulata*	O		X	X	X	X

*The taxonomic nomenclature regarding this animal is under reconsideration for revision.

**The binomial nomenclature for this turtle was formerly *Pseudemys* or *Chrysemys scripta elegans*. It has now been assigned to the genus *Trachemys*.

LEGEND: X = usual food items eaten
M = miscellaneous meats F = fish
FL = flowers, misc. V = other vegetables
FR = fruits

O = occasionally eaten
I/W/S/DF = insects, worms, slugs, snails, *small amounts of dog food*

TABLE 4
FOOD PREFERENCES FOR CROCODILIANS

CROCODILIAN SPECIES	M	FISH	BIRDS	CARRION	FROGS	I
AMERICAN ALLIGATOR *Alligator mississippiensis*	X	X	X	X	X	X
CHINESE ALLIGATOR *Alligator sinensis*	X	X	X	X	X	X
CAIMAN *Caiman sp.; Melanosuchus niger Paleosuchus sp.*	X	X	X	X	X	X
CROCODILE *Crocodylus sp.; Osteolaemus tetraspis*	X	X	X	X	X	X
GAVIAL (GHARIAL) *Gavialis gangeticus*	O	X	O	O	O	O
FALSE GHARIAL *Tomistoma schlegeli*	O	X	O	RARELY	O	O

LEGENDS: X = usual food items   O = occasionally eaten
              M = miscellaneous meats   I = invertebrates/insects

TABLE 5
FOOD PREFERENCES OF THE TUATARA

	INSECTS	IMMATURE MICE	FOWL CHICKS
TUATARA	crickets	X	O
Sphenodon punctatus	silk moth larvae		quail

TABLE 6
COMMON NUTRITIOUS PLANTS
FOR HERBIVOROUS REPTILES

Alfalfa: fresh, sun-cured hay, dried leaves, pellets, meal

Apple: fresh, with peel, sliced or grated (discard core and seeds)

Barley: freshly sprouted seeds, freshly grown leaves, sun-cured hay

Beans (several edible varieties): fresh leaves and stems, fruit; fresh whole, or mashed after soaking in water overnight

Bean sprouts (azuki, black-eyed, garbanzo, lentil, mung, pea, etc.): fresh leaves, stems, blossoms, fruit

Beet: tops, stems, flowers, grated roots

Berseem (Egyptian clover): leaves, sun-cured hay

Brassica species (bok choy, Brussels sprouts, head and Napa cabbage, collards, kale, mustard greens, rape [canola], rutabaga, turnip): fresh green leaves, flowers

Buffalo grass (*Bulbilis dactyloides*): hay

Cactus: flowers, prickly pears, tender young cactus pads

Carrot: leaves, grated root

Clover (Ladino, Alsike, etc.): fresh, sun-cured hay

Corn (maize): kernels

Cotton: leaves, dried or fresh

Cowpea: sun-cured hay, leaves

Cruciferous vegetables: =syn. with *Brassica* sp.; see above

Dandelion: leaves and stems, flowers, fresh or dried

Dicondra: fresh or sun-cured hay

Escarole: fresh leaves

Eugenia: fresh leaves, fruits
Figs: fresh
Grass clippings: freshly mowed or sun-cured
Hibiscus: leaves, flowers, fresh pods
Kudzu: sun-cured hay
Lespedeza: sun-cured hay, leaves
Millet: leaves, sun-cured hay
Mint: sun-cured hay
Mixed vegetables: frozen, thawed
Mulberry: freshly picked tender leaves, fruit
Nasturtium: leaves, stems, flowers
Okra: fresh, chopped, tender leaves and blossoms
Pea: fresh pods, sun-cured hay
Peanut: sun-cured hay with or without nuts
Pear: fresh, cut or grated (discard core and seeds)
Peavine: sun-cured hay
Pelleted commercial chows (Purina, Wayne, etc.) for guinea pigs and rabbits can be fed ad lib; those formulated for horses, goats, dogs, cats or monkeys, etc. SHOULD NOT BE FED IN EXCESS ($< 5\%$ of total diet)
Potentilla ground cover: leaves and blossoms; used as a browse
Saltbush (winter range): sun-cured hay
Soybean: fresh leaves or sun-cured hay
Squash: freshly grated flesh, blossoms, tender leaves
Stone fruits (pitted): apricot, cherry, nectarine, peach, plum, etc.
Sunflower: seeds (unsalted)
Timothy: sun-cured hay
Tofu soybean cake
Triticale: freshly sprouted seeds, sun-cured hay

Vetch: sun-cured hay
Wandering Jew (*Zebrina pendula*): leaves and tender stems
Wheat (soft wheat berries): freshly sprouted, hydroponically grown as a grass

Note that iceberg lettuce, bananas, tomatoes, cucumbers, spinach, Swiss chard, and other calcium-poor, phosphorus-rich, or oxalate-containing plants are not recommended for herbivorous species.

TABLE 7
FOOD VALUES

FOOD	MEASURE	VITAMINS A units	B-1 (mg)	B-2 (mg)	C (mg)	MINERALS CALC. (mg)	PHOS. (mg)	IRON (mg)	OTHER PROT. (gm)
apple	1 small	90	.360	.050	6	7	12	0.3	0
apricot #	3 med.	7,500	.033	.100	4	13	24	0.6	1
asparagus	8 stks	1,100	.360	.065	20	21	40	1.0	2
avocado	1/2 med	500	.120	.137	9	44	42	6.3	2
banana	1 med.	300	.045	.087	10	8	28	0.6	1
beans, grn *	3/4 cup	950	.060	.100	8	55	50	1.1	2
beet greens*	1/2 cup	22,000	.100	.500	50	94	40	3.2	2
beets	1/2 cup	50	.041	.037	8	28	42	2.8	2
blackberries	3/4 cup	300	.025	.030	3	32	32	0.9	2
blueberries	3/4 cup	35	.045	.031	11	25	20	0.9	0
broccoli flr	3/4 cup	6,500	.120	.350	65	64	105	1.3	2
broccoli leaf	3/4 cup	30,000	.120	.687	90	262	67	2.3	3
broccoli stem	3/4 cup	2,000	–	.187	–	83	35	1.1	2
brussels spr	3/4 cup	400	.180	.090	130	27	121	2.1	4
cabbage (1)	1 cup	0	.780	.075	50	46	34	2.0	2
cabbage (2)	1 cup	160	.090	.150	50	429	72	2.8	2
cabbage (3)	1 cup	5,000	.036	.462	50	400	72	2.5	2
cantaloupe	1/2 small	900	.090	.100	50	32	30	0.5	1
carrots (4)	1/2 cup	4,500	.070	.075	5	45	41	0.6	1

cauliflower	3/4 cup	10	.085	.090	75	122	60	0.9	2
celery (5)	4 stlk	20	.030	.015	5	78	46	0.5	1
celery, grn	4 stlk	640	.030	.045	7	98	46	0.8	1
celery root	1/2 cup	—	—	—	2	47	71	0.8	3
chard, lvs*	1/2 cup	15,000	.450	.165	37	150	50	3.1	2
cherries #	12 lrg	259	.051	—	12	19	30	0.4	1
collards *	1/2 cup	6,300	.130	.055	70	207	75	3.4	3
corn on cob	1 med.	860	.209	.054	8	8	103	0.4	3
cucumber	1 med.	35	.060	.270	12	10	21	0.3	1
dandelion grn*	1/2 cup	20,000	.190	.036	100	84	35	0.6	3
eggplant	1/2 cup	70	.042	.072	10	11	31	0.5	1
endive	10 stks	15,000	.058	.060	20	104	39	1.2	3
grapefruit	1/2 med.	20	.070	.024	45	21	20	0.2	1
grapes	1 sm bnch	25	.030	.105	3	19	35	0.7	0
guavas	1	200	.156	—	125	15	16	3.0	1
honeydew mel	1/4 med.	100	—	—	90	—	—	—	0
huckleberry	1/2 cup	100	.045	.021	8	25	20	0.2	1
kale*	1/2 cup	20,000	.189	.570	96	195	67	2.5	4
kohlrabi	1/2 cup	—	.030	.120	50	195	60	0.7	2
leeks	1/2 cup	20	.150	—	24	58	56	0.6	2
lettuce, grn	10 lvs	2,000	.075	.150	7	49	28	1.5	1
lettuce, wht	1/4 head	125	.051	.062	5	17	40	0.5	1
mushrooms (6)	3/4 cup	0	.160	.070	2	14	98	0.7	4
mustard gr.	1/2 cup	11,000	.138	.450	126	291	84	9.1	2
okra	1/2 cup	440	.126	—	17	72	62	2.1	2
onions, frsh	4 med.	60	.042	.125	7	41	47	0.4	1
orange	1 med.	190	.090	.075	50	44	18	0.4	0

FOOD	MEASURE	VITAMINS A (units)	B-1 (mg)	B-2 (mg)	C (mg)	MINERALS CALC. (mg)	PHOS. (mg)	IRON (mg)	OTHER PROT. (gm)
parsley	1/2 cup	8,000	.057	—	70	23	15	9.6	20
parsnips (6)	1/2 cup	100	.120	—	40	60	76	1.7	2
peaches, wht	3 halves #	100	.025	.065	6	10	19	0.2	1
peaches, yel	1 lrg #	1,000	.025	.065	9	10	19	0.3	1
pear	1 med.	17	.030	.060	4	15	18	0.3	0
peas, fresh*	1/2 cup	1,500	.390	.250	20	28	127	0.2	7
persimmon (7)	1 lrg	1,600	—	—	40	22	21	0.2	2
pineapple @	2/3	30	.100	.025	38	8	26	0.2	0
plums	3 med.	130	.120	.056	5	20	27	0.5	1
potato, swt	1 med.	3,600	.155	.150	25	19	45	0.9	3
potato, wht	1 med.	0	.220	.075	33	13	53	1.5	3
potato, yam	1 med.	5,000	.180	.360	6	44	50	1.1	2
pumpkin	1/2 cup	2,500	.056	.057	8	23	50	0.9	2
radishes	15 lg	0	.030	.054	25	21	29	0.9	1
raspberries	1/2 cup	260	.021	—	30	41	38	0.8	1
rutabaga	3/4 cup	25	.075	.120	26	74	56	0.7	1
spinach*	1/2 cup	11,000	.090	.312	30	78	46	2.5	2
squash, hubd	1/2 cup	4,000	.050	.075	3	19	15	0.5	1
squash, sum.	1/2 cup	1,000	.040	.050	3	18	15	0.3	1
strawberries	1/2 cup	100	.025	—	50	34	28	0.6	1
tangerine	2 med.	300	.120	.054	48	42	17	0.2	1

tomatoes	1 med.	1,500	.100	.050	25	11	29	0.4	1
turnips*	1/2 cup	0	.062	.062	22	56	47	0.5	1
turnip grns	1/2 cup	11,000	.060	.045	130	347	49	3.4	2
watercress	3/4 cup	1,250	.030	.090	15	40	11	0.8	0
watermelon	1 med sl	450	.180	.084	22	33	9	0.6	0

LEGEND: (1) inside white leaves   (4) diced   # pitted
         (2) outside green leaves (5) bleached   * cooked
         (3) Chinese   (6) domestic   @ fresh
                           (7) Japanese

Modified from *International Turtle and Tortoise Society Journal*, August/September/October, 1970.

CHAPTER 3

CLINICAL LABORATORY SAMPLE COLLECTION AND PROCESSING

Clinical herpetological animal practice presents many minor and major problems unique to the reptiles and amphibians that comprise this veterinary specialty. Several of these problems involve the techniques for collection and initial processing of specimens that are destined for intramural examination within the clinic setting or for shipment to established clinical laboratories. The following information provides basic and applied techniques that are readily accomplished within the average animal hospital or clinic setting.

In most metropolitan areas, the choice of a clinical veterinary laboratory can be made from one or more accredited commercial sources. In those locales which are not served by one or more daily courier pickups, the clinician may depend upon mail or commercial express services to send specimens to a veterinary clinical laboratory and receive the results by facsimile phone. A local accredited clinical laboratory established for physicians is an alternative. The fee structures of each type of laboratory are often similar and, in some instances, the laboratory geared toward human medicine, even with its typical third-party payment system, may charge less than a solely veterinary lab. Some laboratories have been established for highly specialized submissions.

For instance, diagnostic herpetological histopathology is available from at least three pathologists in the United States who possess the expertise and an interest in herpetofauna. In addition, chemical and physical analysis of urinary, gallbladder, alimentary, and salivary calculi can be obtained at reasonable cost from a highly specialized facility in Massachusetts (Laboratory for Stone Research, Newton, MA).

In order to maximize the usefulness of clinical pathology, the specimens must be obtained correctly, prepared with care, handled gently, fixed by the most appropriate fixative, and packed so that shipping will not make them unusable. Because the costs for diagnostic laboratory analyses are rising steadily, taking a few moments to gather, prepare, handle, identify, and ship specimens properly is cost-effective and will prove to be well worth the effort.

The specimens discussed are skin, blood, bone marrow, urine, feces, gastric lavage samples, sputum and other respiratory samples, semen, materials for microbiological culture (including aerobic, anaerobic, fungal, and virological) and antibiotic sensitivity testing, cerebrospinal fluid, biopsy, exfoliative cytologic, and necropsy tissue samples for routine histopatholgical and electronmicroscopic investigation, toxicological specimens, and ecto- and endoparasites. For purposes of convenience, in those instances where one type of specimen is processed for more than a single examination, it is mentioned separately. In those cases where the test can be accomplished within the clinic setting, specific instructions are provided.

SKIN

(1) Ectoparasites:

Mites can be lifted gently from the host's skin most easily by touching them with a saliva- or water-moistened wooden applicator stick; generally, a cotton-tipped applicator is not used because of the tendency for the parasites to become entangled in the tiny cotton fibers; also, these fibers tend to shed and spoil the finished microscopic whole mount for photography. Ticks should be either pulled off with a forceps, or scraped from the host's integument with a #15 Bard scalpel blade, taking care to remove the entire organism. Transfer mites and ticks to AFA (acid-formalin-alcohol) solution or Pampel's solution* for killing and fixation; they maybe mounted permanently by imbedding them in Hoyer's mounting medium# or Canadian balsam@ beneath a thin coverslip. Gently warming the finished preparation for 12–24 hours at approximately 37–40° clears most mites, small ticks, and lice, and helps disperse entrapped air bubbles. Examine the mounted slide microscopically and, if necessary, identify the specimen taxonomically with the aid of a key to morphological features. Label the slide with the host from which the parasites were recovered, the date, and the taxonomic identification of the parasite. Temporary mounts can be made by using glycerin and water in lieu of Hoyer's medium, but they can be used only for a very brief time. Bulk storage of small ectoparasites can be accomplished by immersing the specimens in a volume of 70% ethanol; thus stored, they may be kept indefinitely.

*, #, see appendix for formulae
@ see appendix for addresses of supplier

(2) Superficial skin mounts:

Remove a small area of affected integument by scraping or snipping off a few scales or scutes with a sterile fine-pattern curved iris scissors and a pair of Adson-Brown forceps, and clear the specimen beneath a coverslip on a slide with mineral oil and xylene, 10% potassium hydroxide, lactol phenol and cotton blue, or other agent to render them transparent and, thus, reveal the presence of ectoparasites, fungi, or other pathogen when viewed microscopically. Warming the preparation at 37–40°C for about 10 minutes accelerates clearing.

In order to identify specific classes of microorganisms prior to culture, stain moist skin exudates directly with Giemsa, acid-fast, PAS, Brown and Brenn's modification of Gram's stain.

(3) Microbiology:

Place similar specimens of skin, scales, or dermal scutes onto DTM fungal growth medium containers and/or onto Sabouraud's fungal culture dishes or vials. Often, subculturing on one or more media enhances the likelihood for a positive isolation. Similarly, place bacterial cultures into transport medium or directly onto blood agar from which subcultures can be made. In most cases, subculturing in thioglycholate-containing medium improves the results because it increases the growth of Gram-negative microorganisms while inhibiting the growth of Gram-positive bacteria.

BLOOD

Blood is obtained from reptiles from a variety of locations and by several methods. When selecting the method for obtaining a specimen, the size of the patient is as important as the volume requirements of the particular test. **DO NOT WITHDRAW MORE BLOOD THAN IS NECESSARY**. Fortunately, the advent of microtechniques permit the clinician and animal health technician to obtain a small, yet adequate, volume of blood from which a large amount of information can be gleaned. For your convenience, I have included a Vacutainer-type collection vial cap color code, consisting of the reagents contained in the vials, in the appendix at the end of this chapter.

In the case of small lizards, snakes, and tiny turtle hatchlings, a few drops to as much as 0.10 ml of whole blood can be drawn without endangering the life of these diminutive patients. From this small amount of blood, the total protein (TP), white cell count (WBC), differential white count, and microscopic examination for cellular abnormalities and hemoparasites, erythrocyte indices (packed cell volume [PCV], hemoglobin concentration, mean corpuscular volume (MCV), mean corpuscular hemoglobin concentration (MCHC), icterus index, and some clinical chemistry tests can be determined. With a slightly larger volume, a full chemistry panel can be obtained. Even a single large drop will yield enough blood for a thin coverslip blood film, PCV measurement (and, thus, estimate of icterus) and glucose determination.

Various techniques have been reported for obtaining blood samples from reptiles. Direct cardiocentesis and venipuncture employing the ventral and lateral caudal veins, jugular, brachial, popliteal, periorbital, pterygo-palatine, and dorsal post-occipital sinuses can be used, depending upon the species and size of the animal.

Toenail clipping has been recommended in both very small and very large captive reptiles. However, in tiny reptiles, the volume of freely flowing blood may be inadequate to accomplish many tests; conversely, in the very large giant tortoises or crocodilians, the efforts required to halt bleeding after the specimens have been obtained may require heroic measures. For this reason, direct venipuncture into a vein or venous sinus is preferred.

Venipuncture into the pterygo-palatine-pharyngeal veins that course longitudinally along the ventromedial surface of the palate of snakes has been described. This method may be useful, but the effort to restrain the snake, open its mouth, enter the veins, and gather an adequate sample may impose an unacceptable stress that often outweighs any potential benefits.

Most turtles, tortoises, and crocodilians possess large paired thin-walled venous sinuses that are immediately caudal to the occipital region. Direct an appropriate-size needle blindly into the area of these sinuses, and withdraw a sufficient volume of blood. Bennett (1986) described this technique in hatchling sea turtles and it is the preferred method for venipuncture in many chelonians and crocodilians.

Enter the orbital vasculature forming the peribulbar and retro-bulbar plexi of small lizards by gently inserting a heparinized microhematocrit tube between the eyelids and direct it to the inner edge of the orbit. By rotating the glass tube, capillaries and arterioles are minimally, yet sufficiently, traumatized to yield a few drops of blood. Then permit the blood to flow up into the lumen of the tube by capillary action. Excessive bleeding is very rare with this technique. Occasionally, the blood specimen may be slightly diluted with the epithelial cells and serous secretions from the periorbital glands, thus yielding an erroneously low packed cell volume and other erythrocyte indices. The extent to which the blood is diluted can be judged by viewing the blood as it is drawn into the microcapillary tube; if blood is interspersed with clear fluid, the results must be adjusted accordingly.

Direct cardiocentesis into the large single ventricle is not only one of the simplest methods but, because of its relative ease, may be one of the safest in small reptiles. In even the smallest snakes, the apical heartbeat can be seen when the snake is placed upon its back and the cranial third of the body is viewed from an angle. Having incident light directed from one side, rather than perpendicularly from above, will aid in seeing the beat. A hand-held transilluminator may help. Prepare the chosen site as for aseptic surgery. Direct a tuberculin or insulin syringe fitted with a 25- to 30-gauge needle into the ventricle, and draw the sample by *gentle* traction on the plunger. Generally, a single cardiocentesis is sufficient; if success is not achieved after one or two attempts, another method should be employed to avoid lacerating the pericardium and/or myocardium.

If, for some reason, the postoccipital venous sinuses or other major veins cannot be employed for venipuncture in chelonians, cardiocentesis can be accomplished through a small hole drilled in the plastron where it covers the ventricle. A landmark for this site is where the ventral midline suture intersects the posterior suture of the pectoral plates. A small sterilized twist drill or Steinmann intramedullary pin can be employed for drilling the hole. After obtaining the specimen with a needle and syringe, cover the plastral hole with epoxy resin, dental acrylic compound, or a few drops of New Skin(R) antiseptic liquid bandage-(Medtech Laboratories, Jackson, WY 83001 USA). Larger turtles and tortoises may be bled readily from their jugular, brachial, popliteal, or caudal vasculature.

The ultrasonic Doppler blood flow detector model 8 (EMS Products, Inc. 1130 8th Street, Kirkland, WA 98033 USA) or models 802-A, 811, and 812 fitted with a pediatric flat probe (Parks Medical Electronics, Inc., P.O. Box 5669, Aloha, OR 97006 USA), greatly facilitate the location of arteries; accompanying veins usually course alongside these muscular vessels. I prefer the EMS instruments because they are very compact, are state-of-the-art, and cost no more than the less compact Parks models. A thin film of water-soluble coupling gel or lubricating jelly is used to enhance the contact between the Doppler's transducer and the patient's integument.

The use of anticoagulants such as sodium or lithium heparin or EDTA (disodium versenate; sequestrene; versene) is dictated by the specific test and the laboratory's protocol and the conditions under which the specimen is drawn. EDTA is contraindicated for specimens destined for calcium ion determinations and tends to induce hemolysis, especially in chelonian erythrocytes. Under field (or zoo) conditions, the time from obtaining the specimen to its delivery to a laboratory may be prolonged, and some form of anticoagulant must be employed to preserve the blood. Lithium heparin anticoagulants seem to meet most requirements for preventing coagulation and preserving cellular morphology.

Blood films should be made as thin as practicable and quickly air-dried. Some clinicians and animal health technicians prefer to make their blood films on coverslips; others use standard glass microscopic slides. Both have their advantages: the cover slip films tend to be thinner, require much less staining reagent, but require much more care to prevent their breakage if they must be mailed; microscope slides are sturdier and are much easier to pack and ship.

When a concentration of leukocytes is desired, make a smear from the buffy coat at the top of the solid cell column of an anticoagulant-coated centrifuged microhematocrit tube. The air-dried smear should be immediately flooded with absolute methanol for more thorough fixation. These techniques will help assure the preservation of not only the blood cells' morphology, but also any hemoparasites, bacteria, or crystalline substances that may be present. Moreover, methanol fixation helps preserve the quality of the slides during transit from the field or animal quarters. After the slides have been identified appropriately, the methanol-fixed blood films will remain in excellent condition if stored in dry dust-proof plastic slide boxes or mailers that prevent them from touching each other. Using slides made with a frosted identification block on one end facilitates identification of each specimen.

Blood drawn for chemical analysis should be separated into serum or plasma and the formed elements before shipping to the clinical laboratory. By doing so, the specimen will be more free of hemoglobin and, thus, will yield more accurate colorimetric values. Blood specimens destined for blood sugar analysis must be submitted in grey-topped tubes so that cellular respiration is halted. Fluid specimens should be protected from shock and breakage, as well as temperature extremes; styrofoam or plastic bubble-wrap achieve both goals and are light weight.

BONE MARROW

Bone marrow is sampled according to the nature and size of the animal patient. Large lizards, crocodilians, and some chelonians yield adequate bone marrow specimens from their femoral marrow cavities. Bone marrow from other chelonians can be sampled by drilling a small hole into the diplöe-like cancellous bone that is sandwiched between the outer and inner layers of the bony shell. This hole is not drilled completely through the shell's thickness but, rather, only through the outer layer. To obtain the specimen, insert a Vim-Silverman[R] (Becton-Dickinson Primary Care Diagnostics, Franklin Lakes, NJ 07417 USA) or similar type biopsy needle into the marrow-bearing cancellous bone, and use a syringe to *gently* aspirate a plug of cells. It is essential to apply only modest vacuum when aspirating the specimen because some of the marrow cells, particularly the multinucleated osteoclast-like precursors of thrombocytes, are exquisitely fragile. Similar care must be taken when distributing the specimen onto a glass slide. If a plug of reasonably solid marrow is obtained, it may be used to make touch impressions rather than the more common method of creating squash-type smears. The touch preparations will yield a higher percentage of intact cells and will better preserve the morphology of all cellular bone marrow elements.

The touch preparations or smears should be air-dried and methanol-fixed (unless the laboratory requests unfixed specimens for some test protocols).

After obtaining the marrow specimen, patch the hole with epoxy or acrylic resin. Large snakes will yield bone marrow from the marrow cavities within their many ribs. The bone marrow of smaller snakes can be sampled by either of two methods: (1) a rib may be excised and fixed in 10% neutral buffered formalin and then decalcified in 15% formic acid solution (or other decalcifying solution) until it is sufficiently soft to permit processing by histological methods; or (2) a biopsy needle can be directed, under radiographic viewing, into the ventral vertebral bodies which contain within their centers sufficient marrow for analysis. The first method may be more appropriate under most conditions; it is safe and effective and yields excellent specimens.

STAINING

For rapid screening of blood films, new methylene blue or a similar product is adequate but, alas, the slides stained by this agent must be destained and then restained and coverslipped if they are to be kept for later examination. There are several excellent rapid stains that will yield splendid results and, if the slides are properly coverslipped and stored, they can be kept for years with little or no degradation of stained cell quality. Almost any Romanowsky-type stain is satisfactory for staining reptilian blood cells. Some of these stains vary only in their buffering requirements and the time required for complete staining. Each hematologist seems to prefer one or another; for those slides which merit photomicroscopic archiving and/or long-term specimen storage, the author has found Kleineberger-Noble's Giemsa to be unsurpassed—but the technique requires 24 hours. The technique of Jenner-Giemsa yields nearly equal results and can be completed in a few minutes. Both of these staining techniques have the decided advantage that slides retained for archival purposes remain beautifully colored for many years if they are stored properly; smears stained with some of the rapid-type staining products may be very nicely colored when freshly stained, but tend to fade even when coverslipped and stored under optimum conditions. For screening purposes, either Diff-Quik(R) (American Scientific Products, Inc., McGaw Park, Il, 60085) or Dip-Stat(R) (Medi-Chem, Inc., Santa Monica, CA, 90404) is satisfactory. The stained specimen is then coverslipped using a permanent mounting medium, or examined with an oil immersion lens without coverslipping. If permanently mounted, allow the coverslip to remain in place over the drop of mounting medium and, after a few moments, use a flat-ended applicator stick to firmly depress the coverslip, and displace any trapped air bubbles. For best results, the stained slide should be dipped in xylene just before applying the mounting medium; this will facilitate even distribution of the medium and improve the quality of the finished specimen. *Note*: if you have identified the slide(s) with an indelible marking pen such as a Sharpie Fine Point(R) permanent marker (Sanford), coat the identification by swiping it with a chemical-soaked Polaroid(R) squeegie that is furnished with black and white Polaroid film packs. Often, these chemically treated devices can be obtained free from imaging laboratories or any other end-user of Polaroid black and white film packs; these squeegies will last for years if they are kept stored in their original cylindrical containers. Allow the chemical coating to dry for several minutes before immersing the treated slide into any xylene-containing solvent.

Stained slides should be kept in slotted slide storage boxes in a relatively cool and dark environment. They should be periodically inspected for evidence of drying of the mounting medium. If medium drying and shrinkage are noticed, the affected slides should be soaked in xylene-toluene until the cover slip falls away from the slide. The slide may then be recoverslipped and, after the new mounting medium has dried, returned to its correct slot in the storage box.

A series of cell-specific stains is now available. These products are highly cell selective and are marketed by Cytocolor, Inc., P. O. Box 401, Hinckley, OH 44233. They are called Lymphocolor(R), which is used to differentiate various lymphocytic cells in blood and bone marrow; Granulocolor(R), which distinguishes the various granulocytes; Neutrocolor(R), designed to identify azurophils; Megacolor(R), which specifically stains megakaryocyte-like cells in bone marrow specimens; Lysocolor(R), which stains lysosomes in some granulocytic cells; and Panoptikon(R), which vividly stains the nuclear chromatin, nucleoli, and cytoplasmic granules found in several cell types. These tinctorial products permit individual acidophilic eosinophils and heterophils, azurophilic neutrophils, and basophils to be distinguished with absolute certainty. If these cell-selective stains are to be used, *DO NOT FIX THE SMEARS WITH METHANOL*.

Microhematocrit tubes should be filled and centrifuged so that the serum or plasma column can be examined for the presence of an abnormal color. The most common abnormalities seen are icteric and hemoglobin-colored fluid, but bright blue and green serum have also been seen. Interestingly, some snakes whose serum or plasma is bright blue or green have been entirely normal, and the underlying cause(s) for the abnormal hues remains unclear.

URINE

Although many terrestrial reptiles produce solid urate-rich urinary wastes, some possess urinary bladders in which the urine is further concentrated by osmotic absorption of water across the bladder wall. Snakes do not possess urinary bladders, although a pseudobladder has been found in at least one snake whose testicular tumor had exerted sufficient extramural pressure to cause the formation of a false bladder from the dilated ureter. Seven urinary calculi were found within this abnormal urinary structure.

If fresh urates cannot be obtained from the cage or enclosure, often it is possible to obtain fresh urine or urates via transcutaneous paracentesis with or without the aid of ultrasonographic imaging. Attempts to pass a catheter from the cloacal vault into the urodeum assume a risk of inducing an ascending urinary tract infection. In larger reptiles, the urodeal ostia can be visualized with the aid of an endoscope, but the risk of carrying fecal bacteria into the urodeum is ever-present. Trying to express urine by compressing the thin-walled bladder through the caudal body wall is not recommended. Because of their microcrystalline nature, solid urates are of minimal value from the standpoint of clinical diagnosis. However, if bile-staining or blood are seen, they may reflect disease. In snakes and lizards, bile-staining may indicate hepatic infection with amoebae and/or trematodes; a piece of green-stained urates mixed with Ringer's or physiologic saline, then coverslipped and examined microscopically may reveal amoebic cysts and/or operculated fluke ova. Usually, amoebic trophozoites are not found in the stools or urates.

Aquatic reptiles and some amphibians produce fluid urine which can be sampled via paracentesis. Many anuran amphibians will voluntarily void urine as a defensive behavior when they are handled; this urine can be caught in a suitable container. SediStain(R) (Becton Dickenson Primary Care Diagnostics, Franklin Lakes, NJ 07417 USA) is as effective in identifying cells in herpetofaunal patients as it is in mammals.

Multistix(R) (Miles Inc. Diagnostics Division, Elkhart IN 46515 USA) are useful for evaluating fluid urine of reptiles just as they are in mammalian patients, and the technique for their use is identical. For more precise measurement of blood glucose, the use of an Accu-Check II M(R) (Boehringer Mannheim Diagnostics Division Indianapolis, IN 46250 USA) or similar device is recommended.

In some instances, azotemic reptiles and amphibians can be identified by the use of Azostix(R) (Miles Inc. Diagnostics Division, Elkhart IN 46515 USA) moistened with either whole blood or coelomic fluid. Some uremic turtles and tortoises exude clear nitrogen-rich fluid from between loosened shell plates. This fluid often yields a strongly positive reaction when applied to the Azo-stix.

Urinary calculi are relatively common occurrences in terrestrial chelonians and some lizards. Most of these stones are composed of varying amounts of sodium- or potassium ammonium urates.

FECES

The specimen of feces should be as fresh as possible. If it is not obtained from the cage, often it can be removed from the terminal alimentary tract by either gentle palpation or by insertion of a fecal extractor or cotton-tipped applicator stick through the cloacal vent. If feces must be sent to an outside laboratory, they should be preserved in polyvinyl alcohol and, ideally, refrigerated.

In-house techniques that are practical for evaluation of feces are: gross examination for the presence of metazoan helminths, microscopic examination of direct smears with and without special staining techniques, floatation and sedimentation specimens, special staining for the presence of protozoan parasites and cloacal mites, special tests for the presence of fecal hemoglobin originating from gastrointestinal bleeding, screening for the presence or absence of pancreatic enzymes, and microbiological culture. Most of these tests are most efficient when applied to fresh feces.

Make direct smears by mixing a small amount of feces with physiologic saline or Ringer's solution, and coverslipping. After the initial examination, add a drop or two of merthiolate or Mayer's hematoxylin to the edge of the coverslip and permit it to diffuse into the fecal specimen. This technique will immediately immobilize and kill any motile microorganisms, thus making them easier to observe and identify. Trichrome stain is especially useful for characterizing protozoa, particularly *Giardia* and many ciliates and flagellated amoebae. Acid-fast stain is easily applied, and greatly helps in the identification of *Cryptosporidium*. Another very useful technique is to view the wet-mount specimen under sheared-light illumination which renders the object being examined in a three-dimensional manner. The shearing condenser is readily available for most of the better microscopes and replaces the Abbé conventional substage condenser. In use, the lever shifts the light path to a more tangential course, thus creating a shadowing effect.

Microbiological analyses of reptilian and amphibian feces are identical to those employed in mammals, with the minor exception that the incubation temperature can be somewhat lower. In fact, lower incubation temperatures may enhance the isolation of pathogens adapted to poikilothermic hosts. Gram stain, especially Brown and Brenn's modification, acid-fast, and PAS stains, are useful in identifying bacterial and mycotic pathogens in feces. Cross-polarized illumination is useful in identifying and characterizing mineral crystals and fibers that might have been ingested or formed within the alimentary tract in response to one or more metabolic derangements.

GASTRIC LAVAGE SPECIMENS

Usually employed in the diagosis of cryptosporidosis, gastric lavage is an easily accomplished and very useful technique that is appropriate in the clinic setting. A typical presentation would be a snake with a history of regurgitation within 24–48 hours after swallowing a meal. Usually, a palpably enlarged stomach is present and, often, can be seen as the patient rests upon a solid surface.

A plastic urethral catheter is premeasured by laying it along-side the patient and marking the approximate distance distal from the mouth. Lubricate the tube lightly with either petroleum jelly or water-soluble gel, and advance it into the esophagus and into the stomach; then introduce a modest volume of normal saline with the aid of a syringe attached to the Luer bell at the open end of the catheter. "Flutter" the stomach so as to mix the introduced fluid with the shed gastric mucosal cells. After a few moments of agitation, withdraw the fluid through the catheter and back into the syringe, and concentrate the specimen by centrifugation. Discard the major portion of the supernatant. Resuspend the "button" at the bottom of the centrifugation tube by agitating it, and place a drop or two onto a clean glass microscope slide; air- or heat fix; and stain with acid-fast or other desired staining reagent (merthiolate, trichrome, Lugol's iodine, Gram's, etc.). As with the microscopic examination of fecal specimens, using a sheared light-path condenser enhances the images of tiny microorganisms.

SPUTUM

The major reason for sampling sputum is to determine whether a reptilian patient is infested with protozoan or metazoan parasites, particularly trichomonads, lungworms, and trematodes. Embryonated ova of *Rhabdias* in snakes and *Entomelas* in lizards, and the adults and golden operculated ova of a variety of small flukes are found in the oropharyngeal secretions of infested fish-, amphibian-, and/or reptile-eating snakes. Embryonated pentastomid ova, characterized by their football-shaped multilayered shell containing a single embryo bearing rudimentary limb appendages, are also found occasionally in snakes.

The technique for sampling sputum entails using a cotton-tipped applicator to obtain a specimen. Roll the moistened cotton tip gently across a clean glass microscope slide, then add a drop of Sedi-Stain, merthiolate, or other coloring agent before coverslipping and examining microscopically. *Rhabdias* and *Entomelas* ova are typically elongated and usually contain a single embryo; they are morphologically similar to, or indistinguishable from, the ova of *Strongyloides stercoralis*.

For safety's sake, wear disposable gloves because some of these parasites pose a potential zoonotic hazard.

SEMEN

Seminal fluid can be obtained occasionally from the penis or hemipenis of some male reptiles, but an easier means for gathering useful specimens is from the cloacal vault of freshly mated females. In either instance, introduce a moistened cotton-tipped applicator into the cloacal vent of the females, inverted hemipenis of male snakes or lizards, or the ventral raphe of the penis of male turtles. Electroejaculation has been described in reptiles and may have a place under some special circumstances. Some reptiles, especially snakes, form "vaginal" or cloacal postcopulatory plugs immediately after they have been successfully mated. These plugs are the result of enzymatic activation of cloacal mucus by enzymes present in the semen of the successful male partner.

Whatever the source of the seminal specimen, spread the sample onto a clean microscopic slide by rolling the moistened cotton-tipped applicator gently across the slide, quickly air-dry, fix in absolute methanol, and stain with Geimsa, Diff-Quick, Sedi-Stain, or any Romanowsky-type polychrome staining product. For archival purposes, coverslip as with blood and bone marrow specimens.

MICROBIOLOGICAL SAMPLING

The methods of gathering specimens and the laboratory culture techniques and media used for isolation and characterization are the same for poikilotherms as they are for mammals and birds. As noted earlier in the section on dermatologic specimens, a minor difference between homeothermic and heterothermic medicine is that often the isolation of Gram-negative bacteria can be enhanced by subculting in thioglycholate-containing media, lower incubation temperatures, and oxygen tensions. Generally, microbiological culture at 24–30°C and a reduced oxygen atmosphere are advised because they often promote the growth of facultative and obligate anaerobes. Provide as much information relating to the nature of the clinical problem and specific requests for tests, along with adequate identification of the specimen.

Many herpetofaunal pathogens pose a potential health hazard for humans; these hazards are avoided easily by wearing appropriate protective gloves and a face mask, and by great care in preventing accidental contaminated needle trauma. Whenever possible, regular culturettes or miniculturettes and transport medium are used to preserve microbiological specimens until they can be Gram-stained and inoculated onto appropriate media in the laboratory. In the in-hospital setting, Gram staining, acid-fast, Giemsa, and similar techniques are practical and can yield rapid results while awaiting results of microbiological culture, which may require several days—or in the case of *Mycobacterium*, several weeks. Typically, a series of antibiotic-impregnated test disks are placed on the agar medium so as to identify which antibiotic agents are most effective against a particular pathogen.

Generally, fungal cultures using either DTM-type color indicator medium or Sabauraud's agar plates can be incubated at 26–32°C, rather than the typical 37°C incubator temperature employed in avian and mammalian mycology. As soon as possible, the cultured organisms can be stained with lactol-phenol/cotton blue to establish a taxonomic identification upon which a rational therapy can be planned.

Gather specimens for virological culture aseptically and place them in specific media recommended by the particular laboratory that will be performing the culture. Generally, duplicated samples are frozen and/or placed in a fixative suitable for electronmicroscopy. When properly handled, samples for virological culture can be shipped under refrigeration via any of several express or courier services. If material is to be sent outside of the United States, a specific permit is required by the Department of Agriculture. If the species from which the specimens were obained is listed on CITES or other registry of endangered animals, special permission must be obtained from the U.S. Department of the Interior's Fish & Wildlife Service.

CEREBROSPINAL FLUID

A small volume of cerebrospinal fluid can be aspirated by inserting a small-diameter/short-bevel hypodermic needle into the cisterna magnum. Prepare the operative site as for routine aseptic surgery, then advance the needle gently until it enters the epidural space. Only minimum vacuum is required to withdraw the drop or two of fluid. **DO NOT EXERT EXCESSIVE BACK PRESSURE**. The CSF can be used for making a stained smear and/or for microbiological culture. The techniques for both of these modalities are identical to those used for blood and other body fluids.

TISSUES

Fresh tissue can be obtained from exfoliative cytologic specimens, biopsy of suspected lesions, and necropsy examination. The fates of these samples include intramural cytology of scrapings, swabs, fine-needle squash preparations, stained histologic sections, and electron microscopy. With few exceptions, tissues destined to be sent for histological examination should not be frozen; rather, they must be placed in an appropriate chemical fixative solution—most often 10% neutral buffered formalin. In some instances, the fixative of choice differs and may be Bouins, Karnovsky's, etc. In these cases, inquire at the pathology laboratory and request special instructions. An exception to using chemical fixation is muscle tissue submitted for biopsy; often, this material should be sent in as a fresh, unfixed specimen that is immediately frozen, sectioned, stained, and examined microscopically. Thus, these special cases are best handled after *ADVANCED* planning with a local pathology laboratory equipped to render intraoperative histopathology. Tissues containing suspected urate deposits should be fixed in methanol rather than formalin because the methanol will preserve the integrity of urate microcrystals, whereas formalin will dissolve them. Tissues submitted for electronmicroscopy must be as fresh as possible and cut into tiny blocks approximately 1.0 mm on a side, and placed immediately into cold glutaraldehyde solution. When handling glutaraldehyde, great case must be exercised to avoid contact with unprotected skin, mucous membranes, and corneal epithelium. Thus, protective gloves and eyewear should be worn, and a vacuum hood or other means for adequate ventilation must be used whenever working with an open container of fixative.

Tissues from complete necropsies should include skin, skeletal muscle, a small piece of bone, bone marrow (either as a plug removed from the medullary cavity or included with a rib or other marrow-containing bone), esophagus, stomach, intestine (several pieces from different segments), liver and gallbladder, spleen, pancreas, kidneys, gonads and their associated tubular structures, myocardium, thyroid, parathyroid, and thymus. Sensory organs, brain and spinal cord are submitted, if possible, either *in situ* or removed, as described below.

Tissues containing bone or mineralized foci should be decalcified before they are microsectioned in the laboratory.

Generally, these tissues are formalin-fixed for an adequate time to preserve their architecture, then treated for a period of several hours to several days, depending upon their thickness and/or amount of mineralization. Several commercial decalcification solutions containing mixtures of formic and hydrochloric acid, together with EDTA, are available. Warming the post-fixed tissue that is being decalcified will lessen the time required to soften the specimen sufficiently to permit sectioning without damage to the microtome blade. I have found that using a microwave oven to warm the solution and specimen is an efficient and rapid means for accomplishing this task. Generally warming to approximately 40°C one or more times during a period of an hour is sufficient to decalcify sections 3–5 mm thick. Actual bony tissue containing flinty compact bone may require a day or two to become adequately softened to permit microsectioning.

The brain and spinal cord of small reptiles and amphibians are most conveniently sectioned *in situ*, after adequate formalin fixation and decalcification. This technique will preserve the anatomic relationship and the histologic features of delicate structures that otherwise would be disrupted by conventional removal of these tissues. If you decide to remove the brain and/or spinal cord from within their bone-surrounded locations, use a sharp dental pick and fine-pattern *curved* iris scissors and a pair of Adson-Brown tissue forceps because they will make the task easier while causing less damage to these delicate tissues. Splitting the skull in its mid-sagittal plane with a single-edge razor blade or fine-toothed hacksaw blade often will facilitate the operation and will, at the same time, give access to the pituitary. Remove the mandibles, turn the skull with the oral surface facing upward, and tap the razor blade sharply with a small hammer or mallet to help cut through the bony skull in a single try.

Fix sections of hollow viscus organs such as stomach, intestine, gallbladder, and urinary bladder by either filling the tubular or sac-like structure with 10% neutral buffered formalin or tying off one or both ends so that the fixative remains trapped within. Place the now-distended segment into a sufficient volume of formalin for complete preservation prior to selecting tissues for histologic processing. Another means for preserving the architectural features of mucosae is to incise and open segments, place them onto either glass slides or pieces of wooden tongue blade, and immerse the tissue, along with its flat support device, into 10% buffered formalin. Both techniques yield superior tissue specimens for histologic studies.

When submitting specimens of hollow alimentary organs, be sure to look for and remove pieces of grit or gravel that may have been ingested—they will wreak havoc on the delicate edge of a microtome. An easy way to remove such foreign material is to gently rinse the tissue under a small stream of running water. The histo-technicians working with the tissue that you submit will greatly appreciate your consideration.

Very tiny pieces of tissue should be placed into small vials. (I recycle 1.0 ml vaccine diluent vials by removing the aluminum retaining band around the rubber stopper, rinsing the vials several times in distilled water, and replacing the stoppers. These containers are perfect for holding pituitary and other small glandular structures, small spleens, small lateral and/or parietal eyes, punctate lesions, etc.) Fill the vials with

0.5–1.0 ml of formalin. Once filled, place the vials into the containers holding larger pieces of tissue.

Place containers of tissues in Zip-Loc(R)-like or Whirl-Pak(R) (Nasco) plastic bags to prevent leakage. Once preserved in formalin (or other fixative), the specimens can be shipped without additional fluid; this will greatly lessen the cost of shipment and the tissues will not be harmed. Be certain that whatever container is used, it is leak-free; if in doubt, use an additional Zip-Loc(R) bag or two, or some other form of container making sure that the locking device or lid is secured tightly.

PLEASE NOTE: It requires advanced planning if you wish to submit entire cadavers to a pathologist for necropsy. Nothing is more displeasing to the U.S. Postal Service's minions who deliver and the pathologists who receive an unanticipated and often inadequately refrigerated dead animal on the doorstep—particularly on a Monday after the package and its contents have spent an entire weekend slowly but steadily decomposing! To avoid this situation, (1) plan for a Tuesday through Friday delivery, and (2) pack the cadaver in a styro-foam container with an adequate number of freeze packs to ensure that the entire carcass remains chilled. If you are unable to wait over a weekend or holiday to send the cadaver for necropsy, (1) perform the necropsy yourself and send well selected formalin-fixed tissues, or (2) send the dead beastie by Federal Express, United Parcel Service *Blue Label* service, or Express Mail, and **BE CERTAIN THAT THE RECIPIENT IS EXPECTING YOUR SUBMISSION**. The laboratory may be closed, or the pathologist might be lecturing a half a world away or may be on a well deserved vacation. Without such advanced planning, your precious specimen may self-destruct into an unmentionable and thoroughly loathesome mess. Just as the best vintage wines begin as prime grapes, histopathology requires well preserved tissues.

STOMACH, INTESTINAL CONTENTS, AND WATER FOR TOXICOLOGY

When specimens of gastrointestinal contents or water are to be submitted for toxicological screening and analysis, it is best to select samples and then freeze them in the specimen container chosen by the laboratory to whom they are to be sent. The container must be clean (preferably new), identified with the clinician's name and address, owner's name, nature of the specimen, and test(s) requested. If poisoning is suspected, the original container that held the suspected toxicant should be provided, if still available. Specimens of water should be 50–100 ml to assure that a sufficient volume is available to permit adequate testing.

TRACHEAL AND TRANSTRACHEAL SPECIMENS

Often, the specific diagnosis of respiratory conditions requires cytological and microbiological examination of material obtained directly from the lumen of the trachea, mainstem bronchi, and/or lung(s) of the reptilian patient. Anatomical differences dictate the choice of collections sites and methods. For instance, chelonians, because of their ability to withdraw their heads and necks into their shells, have very short tracheas which immediately bifurcate into twin mainstem bronchi that course along the sigmoid flexure of their elongated necks. Most snakes possess only a single lung and nearly all snakes' lungs terminate in nonrespiratory thin-walled sac-like structures that function as hydrostatic organs.

Because of these and other considerations, it is often more practical to obtain intraluminal respiratory specimens by introducing an appropriate volume of sterile saline or other physiological solution into the trachea through the laryngeal glottis and, after manipulating the animal's posture, aspirating the specimen with the intralaryngeal/intratracheal catheter attached to a syringe. The catheter can be a short vascular, closed-end tomcat, or thin canine (or human) urethral catheter, depending upon the length and diameter required. All have a belled end which will accept the Luer tip of a disposable syringe.

Place the specimen of aspirated fluid into a small centrifuge tube and spin it for at least one minute to concentrate the cellular and debris constituents into a "button" at the bottom of the tube. Withdraw the surplus supernatant fluid, resuspend the button by agitating the tube, place a drop or two onto a clean glass slide, add a drop of SediStain or similar coloring reagent, coverslip, and examine microscopically. If the specimen is to be forwarded to a pathology laboratory for cytologic investigation, request specific instructions because it may be necessary to preserve the specimen with formalin or other tissue fixative.

SPECIMENS FOR PARASITOLOGICAL IDENTIFICATION

Ectoparasites and endoparasites often are submitted for taxonomic identification. Sometimes, this identification can be readily accomplished by the clinical laboratory; other times, the specimens must be forwarded to a regional or national center where there are specialists who possess the necessary expertise to make a definitive diagnosis. This service may require weeks or months to complete, and may involve considerable expense to the person making the request.

It is important that the specimen be properly preserved in a way that will retain the morphological features of the organism. For arthropod ectoparasites, 50–70% ethanol is adequate. For many endoparasitic helminths, AFA (acid-formalin-alcohol) solution, Pampel's fluid# or polyvinyl alcohol are the fixatives of choice. However, these specific fixatives often are not readily at hand; in such cases, one can improvise by mixing vodka with equal volumes of 10% formalin solution and white vinegar. Generally, this home-made substitute will preserve helminths until they can be transferred into a more conventional fixative. Whenever possible, try to keep the specimens in a natural and/or straight position; i.e. avoid coiling them up just to fit into a convenient container.

Be certain to label the specimen(s) with the pertinent information before shipping to the laboratory. Recording the parasites on color film prior to preservation often proves to be a worthwhile precaution.

ADDITIONAL TIPS

When using polypropylene cups with screw-on tops to mail specimens to a laboratory, apply Denison[R]-type pressure-sensitive labels on which the addressee's name and mailing address are typed or printed in *indelible ink* and overlap a length of the label so that the cap will be additionally secured. Leave enough room to affix adequate postage. These pressure-sensitive labels will stick to the otherwise adhesive-resistant plastic surface.

If you know the binomial taxonomic classification of the creature whose tissues or body fluids are being submitted for analysis, be certain to supply that information along with the other pertinent data—it will save the pathologists's valuable time having to do a search and, in providing this vital nomenclature, you will earn the respect that such courtesies deserve. (I have had to waste much time in trying to search for information that could have been supplied very easily by the person requesting diagnostic assistance).

Always provide your full name, address, zip code, telephone (and fax) numbers along with the other clinical information in your request for laboratory work; it is amazing how many people take for granted that such simple data is readily available. Do not assume that you or your clinic are so well known that everyone has them in their Rolodex file.

Most of these recommendations are common-sense, and the clinician familiar with herpetological practice is already aware of them.

Whereas many clinical laboratories can provide the majority of the services that are usually required, not all laboratories employ pathologists or technicians who possess the expertise to recognize the often subtle hematological, parasitological, or histological characteristics that differentiate mammalian and herpetofaunal tissues, or the variations that should be observed as inflammatory or neoplastic processes in reptiles and amphibians. Nor can many clinical laboratories established for human or conventional veterinary medical patients render a taxonomic identification of parasites beyond their broad classification into mites, ticks, nematodes, platyhelminthes, etc. Therefore, I encourage you to establish a cordial and enthusiastic rapport with experts in these ephemerally ecclectic fields—it will be reciprocated to the benefit of all concerned.

APPENDIX

* FORMULA FOR HOYER'S MOUNTING MEDIUM FOR SMALL ARTHROPODS

distilled water	50 parts
gum arabic (teardrop form)	30 "
chloral hydrate	200 "
glycerine U.S.P.	20 "

Dissolve gum arabic in water with chloral hydrate for 24–48 hours; add glycerine; filter and store in tightly stoppered squeeze bottles.

#FORMULA FOR PAMPEL'S FLUID (IMPROVED) FOR PRESERVING ARTHROPODS AND HELMINTHS

formalin, 35–37%	6 parts
ethyl alcohol, 95%	15 "
glacial acetic acid	2 "
distilled water	30 "

Mix and use cold; after 2–3 weeks, remove specimen(s) and transfer to 80% enthanol for long-term storage.

@ Canadian balsam (neutral or mixed with xylene) can be obtained from Carolina Biological Supply Co. In the eastern half of the U.S., the address is Burlington, NC 27215; telephone

1-800-334-5551. In the western half of the U.S. the address is Powell Laboratories Division, Gladstone, OR 97027; telephone 1-800-547-1733.

For more detailed information, please refer to Frye (1991) **BIO-MEDICAL AND SURGICAL ASPECTS OF CAPTIVE REPITLE HUSBANDRY, 2ND ED**. in two volumes. Krieger Publishing Co., Inc., Malabar, FL USA

COLOR CODE CHART FOR BECTON DICKINSON VACUTAINER(R), MONOJECT(R), VENOJECT(R), AND TERUMO(R) BLOOD COLLECTION TUBES

COLOR OF RUBBER STOPPER	PRODUCT DESCRIPTION REAGENT, IF ANY	PURPOSE
RED	EVACUATED TUBE, NO ADDITIVES	SEPARATED SERUM
RED/DARK GRAY BANDS	SST GEL AND CLOT ACTIVATION	SEPARATED SERUM
LAVENDER	LIQUID K^3EDTA or FREEZE-DRIED Na_2 EDTA	COMPLETE BLOOD COUNT
GRAY	POTASSIUM OXALATE/ SODIUM FLUORIDE; or SODIUM FLUORIDE; or LITHIUM IODOACETATE/ LITHIUM HEPARIN	BLOOD GLUCOSE DETERMINATION
LIGHT GRAY/DARK GRAY BANDS	THROMBIN	STAT DETERMINATIONS FOR CHEMISTRIES
LIGHT BLUE	0.105 M SODIUM CITRATE (3.2%) or 0.129 M SODIUM CITRATE (3.8%)	COAGULATION DETERMINATION OF PLASMA
DARK BLUE	SODIUM HEPARIN; or Na_2EDTA; or NONE	TOXICOLOGY TRACE ELEMENTS AND NUTRIENTS
GREEN	NON-SILICONE COATED, LITHIUM HEPARIN; or SODIUM HEPARIN; or AMMONIUM HEPARIN	BLOOD CHEMISTRY; CYTOGENETICS (also used for chelonian hematology)

SAMPLE COLLECTION AND PROCESSING

LIGHT GREEN	ACD SOLUTION A	CYTOGENETICS/ MOLECULAR BIOLOGY
BRIGHT YELLOW	SODIUM POLYETHOLE-SULFONATE (SPS)	BLOOD CULTURE/ MICROBIOLOGY
BROWN	SODIUM HEPARIN	LEAD DETERMINATIONS
BLACK	BUFFERED SODIUM CITRATE	SEDIMENTATION RATE ONLY

Source: Becton Dickenson Vacutainer Systems, Rutherford, NJ 07070 USA
Collection vials fitted with Hemogard closures are similarly colored with the exception of the dark gray mottling which is present only on the rubber stoppers.

TABLE 8
NUMBER OF ERYTHROCYTES PER CUBIC MILLILITER OF BLOOD IN REPTILES

Species	Count	Authority
TESTUDINES		
Chelydra serpentina	154,166–530,000	Gaumer & Goodnight (1957); Hutchinson & Szarski (1965)
Chrysemys p. dorsalis	240,000–755,000	Hutchinson & Szarski (1965)
Chrysemys p. marginata	395,000	Gaumer & Goodnight (1957)
Chrysemys p. picta	370,000–829,000	Hutchinson & Szarski (1965)
Clemmys guttata	475,000–750,000	Hutchinson & Szarski (1965)
Clemmys japonica	442,000	Mori (1940)
Emydoidea blandingii	370,000–625,000	Hutchinson & Szarski (1965)
Emys orbicularis	260,000–680,000	Alder & Huber (1923); Babudieri (1930); Salgues (1937a); Duguy (1967)
*Gopherus agassizii**	550,000	Babudieri (1930)
Malaclemys terrapin	620,000–770,000	Hutchinson & Szarski (1965)
Psammobates geometricus	642,000	Bernstein (1938)
Pseudemys scripta	373,000	Babudieri (1930)
Pseudemys scripta elegans	257,000–835,000	Charipper & Davis (1932); Hutton & Charipper (1932); Kaplan & Rueff (1960)
Pseudemys scripta troostii	495,000	Gaumer & Goodnight (1957)
Sternotherus odoratus	360,000–980,000	Hutchinson & Szarski (1965)

Species	Count	Authority
Terrapene carolina	275,000–740,000	Wintrobe (1933); Gaumer & Goodnight (1957) Altman & Thompson (1958) Altman & Dittmer (1961)
Terrapene carolina major	235,000–755,000	Hutchinson & Szarski (1965)
Testudo graeca ibera	362,000–730,000	Hayem (1879); Babudieri (1930); Salgues (1937a); Peña Roche (1939); Grazoadei (1954); Girod & Lefranc (1958)
Trionyx spinnifer asper	530,000–960,000	Hutchinson & Szarski (1965)
CROCODILIA		
Alligator mississippiensis	618,000 to 1,480,000	Hopping (1923); Wintrobe (1933); Coulson, et al. (1950); Altman & Dittmer (1961)
SAURIA		
Acanthodactylus erythrurus	846,000	Salgues (1937a)
Agama atra	1,250,000	Pienaar (1962)
Anguis fragilis	466,000 to 1,615,000	Alder & Huber (1923); Salgues (1937a); Duguy (1963a)
Chalcides ocellatus	806,000	Babudieri (1930); Salgues (1937a)
Coleonyx variegatus	491,000	Ryerson (1949)
Cordylus giganteus	650,000	Pienaar (1962)
Cordylus vittifer	850,000 to 1,790,000	Pienaar (1962)
Heloderma suspectum	646,000	Ryerson (1949)
Hemidactylus turcicus	866,000	Salgues (1937a)

Species	Count	Authority
Lacerta agilis	945,000 to 1,420,000	Hayem (1879); Alder & Huber (1923); Salgues (1937a); Peña Roche (1939)
Lacerta lepida	1,124,000	Salgues (1937a)
Lacerta muralis	960,000 to 2,050,000	Alder & Huber (1923); Babudieri (1930); Salgues (1937a); Peña Roche (1939); Duguy (1967)
Lacerta viridis	840,000 to 1,600,000	Babudieri (1930); Salgues (1937a); Peña Roche (1939)
Lacerta vivipara	1,132,000	Salgues (1937a)
Liolaemus nigromaculatus	1,320,000 to 1,920,000	Peña Roche (1939)
Liolaemus pictus	1,488,000 to 1,800,000	Peña Roche (1939)
Phrynosoma solare	745,000	Ryerson (1949)
Phyllodactylus europaeus	644,000	Salgues (1937a)
Psammodromus hispanicus	756,000	Salgues (1937a)
Sceloporus magister	1,224,000	Salgues (1937a)
Tarentola mauritanica	692,000 to 842,000	Alder & Huber (1923); Salgues (1937a)
OPHIDIA		
Agkistrodon piscivorus	468,000 to 697,000	Hutton (1958)
Coluber constrictor	730,000 to 1,075,000	Hutton (1958)
Coluber viridiflavus	908,000 to 1,608,000	Babudieri (1930); Salgues (1937a)
Coronella austriaca	580,000 to 1,406,000	Babudieri (1930); Salgues (1937a)
Coronella girondica	1,900,000	Salgues (1937a)
Crotalus horridus	1,140,000	Carmichael & Petcher (1945)

Species	Count	Authority
Elaphe longissimus	622,000 to 1,410,000	Babudieri (1930); Salgues (1937a)
Elaphe quadrivirgata	829,750	Mori (1940)
Elaphe scalaris	1,181,000	Salgues (1937a)
Heterodon contortrix	500,000 to 690,000	Wintrobe (1933); Altman & Dittmer (1961)
Lampropeltis g. getulus	538,000 to 690,000	Hutton (1958)
Malopon monspessulanus	1,442,000	Salgues (1937a)
Natrix maura	378,000 to 1,070,000	Salgues (1937a); Duguy (1967)
Natrix natrix	668,000 to 1,302,000	Hayem (1879); Babudieri (1930); Salgues (1937a)
Natrix sipedon pictiventris	570,000 to 885,000	Wintrobe (1933); Hutton (1958); Altman & Dittmer (1961)
Pituophis catenifer sayi	1,090,000	Ryerson (1949)
Thamnophis sirtalis	710,000 to 1,390,000	Wintrobe (1933); Altman & Dittmer (1961)
Tropidophis pardalis	501,000	Hecht, *et al* (1955)
Vipera ammodytes	667,000	Babudieri (1930)
Vipera aspis	571,000 to 1,410,000	Babudieri (1930); Dastigue & Joy (1941)
Vipera berus	615,000 to 1,232,000	Salgues (1937a)
Vipera ursinii	1,350,000	Salgues (1937a)

*Renamed *Xerobates agassizii*

TABLE 9
LEUKOCYTIC FORMULAE OF VARIOUS SOUTH AFRICAN REPTILES*

Percentages of Types of Leukocytes (Identifiable Precursors Included with Definitive Types of Cells)

GENUS & SPECIES	NO. OF SPECIMENS	EOSINOPHILS	BASOPHILS	AZUROPHILS	NEUTROPHILS	LYMPHOCYTES	MONOCYTES	PLASMA CELLS	PRIMITIVE CELLS	THROMBOCYTES
Geochelone pardalis	1	58.0	4.6	5.2	0.0	29.8	2.0	0.0	0.4	95
Homopus areolatus	1	51.6	3.4	1.6	0.0	42.0	0.4	0.8	0.2	90
Pelomedusa subrufa	1	13.8	15.8	6.0	0.0	62.0	0.0	1.6	0.8	245
Pelosios sinuatus	1	35.6	3.6	4.0	0.0	56.0	0.0	0.4	0.4	190
Agama atra	3	14.3	3.7	3.1	1.4	74.3	0.6	1.6	1.0	65
*Agama atricollis***	1	3.9	1.0	0.9	0.2	89.4	2.4	0.9	1.3	25

Species								
Chamaeleo dilepsis dilepsis	2	23.8	3.6	11.0	0.0	59.6	0.0	1.2	0.8	195
Cordylus giganteus	1	38.8	8.0	13.2	2.6	35.0	0.0	1.2	1.2	80
Cordylus jonesii	2	10.0	26.6	11.4	3.4	45.4	0.0	2.6	0.6	90
Cordylus vittifer	20	13.2	7.2	6.6	3.2	66.8	0.8	0.9	1.3	50
Ichnotropis squamulosa	2	59.9	4.0	15.4	0.0	23.3	0.0	0.8	0.6	300
Lygodactylus c. capensis	5	13.4	15.6	15.0	0.0	50.8	0.0	4.2	1.0	62
Mabuya capensis	1	49.4	12.2	17.8	0.0	17.0	0.0	3.2	0.4	72
Mabuya striata	2	40.8	10.8	21.3	0.0	24.9	0.0	1.2	1.0	88
Mabuya varia	3	34.4	19.0	9.0	0.0	36.6	0.0	0.6	0.4	75
Pachydactylus c. capensis	3	18.6	15.9	23.4	0.0	38.6	0.0	2.3	1.2	45
Pachydactylus bibroni	2	19.5	27.8	6.7	0.0	40.2	0.0	2.9	2.9	165
Varanus niloticus	2	11.3	0.1	10.8	0.0	73.7	0.0	3.1	1.0	130
Albabophis rufulus	2	15.6	17.6	16.0	0.0	49.2	0.0	0.8	0.8	350
Causus rhombeatus	2	12.8	9.2	49.8	8.0	17.2	0.2	2.4	0.4	175
Crotaphopeltis hotamboeia	2	11.0	11.4	22.8	0.0	51.8	0.0	2.4	0.6	155
Naja nigrocollis	1	7.6	0.4	44.8	0.0	44.4	0.0	2.4	0.4	135
Psammophis s. subtaeniatus	1	5.5	26.4	28.7	0.0	36.6	0.0	1.6	1.2	200
Crocodylus niloticus	1	11.1	7.7	6.7	0.0	72.3	0.0	1.6	0.6	70

*Data slightly modified from Pienaar, 1962
**The single Agama atricollis was abnormal, being affected with leukemia or some similar pathologic condition.

While restricted to South African reptiles, this table is included because, to date, Pienaar is the only investigator who has counted absolute numbers of thrombocytes in relation to leukocytes.

TABLE 10
RANGE OF FREQUENCIES OF THE DIFFERENT TYPES OF LEUKOCYTES THROUGHOUT THE YEAR IN REPTILES

SPECIES	AUTHORITY	LYMPHO-CYTES	MONO-CYTES	EOSINO-PHILS	BASO-PHILS	HETERO-PHILS
Vipera aspis	Duguy (1963a)	2%–90%	0–5%	0–75%	0–40%	2%–65%
Natrix maura	Duguy (1967)	4%–87%	0–5%	1%–68%	0–25%	5%–75%
Anguis fragilis	Duguy (1963b)	10%–77%	0–3%	3%–67%	0–28%	4%–62%
Lacerta muralis	Duguy (1967)	45%–96%	0–5%	1%–30%	0–12%	2%–23%
Emys orbicularis	Duguy (1967)	45%–76%	0–1%	12%–89%	0–25%	2%–21%

TABLE 11
SEASONAL CHANGES IN THE LEUKOCYTIC FREQUENCIES OF REPTILES

SPECIES	AUTHORITY	SEASON	LYMPHO-CYTES %	MOMO-CYTES %	EOSINO-PHILS %	BASO-PHILS %	HETERO-PHILS %
Vipera aspis	Duguy (1963a)	Summer	50	1	13	10	26.0
		Winter	6	1	70	8	15.0
Natrix maura	Duguy (1967)	Summer	54	1	19	3	23.0
		Winter	32	1	39	3	25.0
Anguis fragilis	Duguy (1963b)	Summer	54	0.5	23	6	16.5
		Winter	16.5	0	58	2	24.0
Lacerta muralis	Duguy (1967)	Summer	81	1	10	1	7.0
		Winter	47	4	28	5	16.0
Emys orbicularis	Duguy (1967)	Summer	52	0	40	4	4.0
		Winter	11	0	83	0	6.0

TABLE 12
PLASMA ELECTROLYTES

SPECIES	OSMOTIC PRESSURE (mOs/l)	pH	Na+	K+	Ca++	Mg++	Cl–	HCO₃	P₁	SO₄	SOURCE*
			(Mm/l)								
TESTUDINES											
Chelydra serpentina	315	7.62	132	3.2	3.8**	2.7	76	48	1.3	0.3	12,29 40,47
Kinosternon subrubrum	288		121	4.2	3.5**	1.0	98	30	1.7		12,47
Sternotherus odoratus	282	7.44	126	3.8			84	25	1.8		12
Chrysemys picta		7.77	143	3.2	2.5**	4.8	85	47	1.0	0.8	24,47 57,60
Emydoidea blandingii			140	3.8	2.1**		91	39	1.3	1.3	47,57
Emys orbicularis	249							40	2.1		4,37,55
Graptemys geographica			124	2.4	3.4**		87	39	1.2	0.4	47
Pseudemys (Trachemys) scripta		7.56	121	4.1	2.8**	2.2	81	40	1.1	0.2	7,12,24,33, 45,47,50,51
Terrapene carolina	345	7.68	130	4.7	1.3**	3.5	108		2.4	1.2	12,24 34

Species								
Terrapene ornata	317							12
Caretta caretta	408							4,5,18, 19,31,44,47
		157	2.2	1.7**	2.0	104	0.8	
			4.6	3.1**	2.9	110	3.0	
Lepidochelys olivacea		163	6.6	5.2**	1.4	108	3.5	
Chelonia		158	1.5					
mydas		7.45						0.3 47
Chelonia* mydas		172	5.3	9.1	N.D.	113	44**	
Testudo graeca	321		7.8	4.0**		100	6.7	3,31
Testudo hermanni	317	127	4.4	2.3**		95		5,43
Trionyx ferox	274	113	6.8	1.7**	1.5	90	2.0	25
Trionyx spiniferus		144						12
SQUAMATA (Sauria)								22
Gekko gecko						123		12
Anolis carolineneis		7.26	157	4.6	2.9**	127	2.6	12,35
Anolis.			171	4.5				42
Ctenosaura acanthura		7.22	159	2.9	2.9**	1.1	133	2.3	30
Ctenosaura pectinata			171	4.4				49
Iguana iguana		7.48	157	3.5	2.7**	0.9	118	2.0	30,56,58
Sauromalus obesus		7.50	169	4.9			127		16,49
Sceloporus occidentalis					2.5**				41

SPECIES	OSMOTIC PRESSURE (mOs/l)	pH	Na⁺	K⁺	Ca⁺⁺	Mg⁺⁺	Cl⁻	HCO₃	P₁	SO₄	SOURCE*
			(Mm/l)								
Amphibolurus ornatus			150	5.0							61
Agama agama	349		179	5.2							53
Agama impalearis	307		152	7.1	2.9**						59
Uromastyx acanthinurus			150		2.5**						59
Chamaeleo chameleon							114				12
Eumeces fasciatus			130								12
Trachydosaurus rugosus			151	4.7							1,46
Cnemidophorus sexlineatus							128				12
Tupinambis nigropunctatus			136	3.5			110				12
Ophisaurus ventralis	388	7.16									12
Gerrhonotus (Elgaria) multicarinatus	353										12
Heloderma suspectum		7.20					130	27			23

Species									
Heloderma horridum			158	4.1	3.1**	2.3	114		54
Varanus griseus			181	3.5	3.1**	2.3	148	31	2.5	27
SQUAMATA (Ophidia)									
Lichanura roseofusca							106			12
Coluber constrictor	375	7.63	151	4.1	3.2**	1.5	101			13,22
Elaphe obsoleta	384		162	4.9	3.6**	2.5	131		2.5	12
Farancia abacura	313		147	5.4	3.3**		115			12
Heterodon platyrhinos		7.53	155	4.4			126	12		12
Lampropeltis getulus	345	7.46	148	4.5	2.9**	1.9	121	10	2.4	12,32
Masticophis flagellum	341		156	3.9	3.4**	2.1	120		1.1	12
Pituophis catenifer	381		176	5.9	3.6**		136			12
Rhinocheilus lecontei			164	4.1			122			12
Natrix erythrogaster		7.22	192	5.0			146	10		12
Natrix natrix			159	6.4						42
Natrix rhombifera	359	7.32	155	4.0	3.9**		149	7		12
Natrix sipedon	318	7.29	159	4.6	3.8**	1.3	127	11	2.3	10,12,32,38
Regina grahamiae	354		156	3.5	3.8**		120			12
Thamnophis elegans	347	7.20	161	4.3	3.4**	0.8	134	14	1.9	12

SPECIES	OSMOTIC PRESSURE (mOs/l)	pH	Na+ (Mm/l)	K+	Ca++	Mg++	Cl−	HCO3	P1	SO4	SOURCE*
Thamnophis ordinoides	349	7.27	159	5.4			126	10			12
Thamnophis sauritus	324	7.19	159	5.4	2.7**	2.0	125	14	1.6		12,13
Thamnophis sirtalis	329	7.30	152	5.9	3.0**	1.5	130		0.7		12,14
Homalopsis buccata			162	4.8	4.2**						2
Micrurus fulvius							134				12
Agkistrodon contortrix	361	7.32	154	5.1	3.5	2.3	138	12			12
Agkistrodon piscivorus	401		151	5.0	3.4	1.7	116	10	1.8		12,32
Crotalus atrox	345		154	3.7	3.7	1.8	131				12,39
Crotalus horridus							112				6
Crotalus viridis	325		146	3.6			123				12
Vipera aspis			170	6.5	3.5		130		3.5		11,36
Laticauda semifasciata	320		159								21
CROCODILIA											
Alligator mississippiensis	284	7.46	141	3.8	2.6**	1.5	112	20			8,9,17
Crocodylus acutus			149	7.9	3.4	1.9	117	11			15

* values obtained from juvenile wild turtles
** ion balance (Na − (Cl + CO_2)

*Numbers designate reference sources listed below (cited in Frye, 1991)
**These data appear in the light of more recent determinations, less than normal and may reflect the laboratory methodology employed.

1. Bentley, 1959
2. Bergman, 1951
3. Berkson, 1966
4. Bottazzi, 1908
5. Burian, 1910
6. Carmichael & Petcher, 1945
7. Collip, 1921a,b; 1920
8. Coulson & Hernandez, 1964
9. Coulson, et al. 1950a
10. Dantzler, 1967
11. Dastugue & Joy, 1943
12. Dessauer, unpublished, 1952
13. Dessauer & Fox, 1959
14. Dessauer, et al. 1956
15. Dill & Edwards, 1931
16. Dill & Edwards, 1935
17. Dill, et al. 1935
18. Drilhon & Marcoux, 1942
19. Drilhon, et al. 1937
20. Dunlap, 1955
21. Dunson & Taub, 1967
22. Dunson & Weymouth, 1965
23. Edwards & Dill, 1935
24. Gaumer & Goodnight, 1957
25. Gilles-Baillien & Schoffeniels, 1965
26. Grollman, 1927
27. Haggag, et al. 1965
28. Haning & Thompson, 1965
29. Henderson, 1928
30. Hernandez & Coulson, 1951
31. Holmes & McBean, 1964
32. Hutton, 1958
33. Hutton, 1960
34. Hutton & Goodnight, 1957
35. Hutton & Ortman, 1957
36. Izard, et al. 1957
37. Laskowski, 1936
38. LeBrie & Sutherland, 1962

39. Luck & Keeler, 1929
40. McCay, 1931
41. Mullen, 1962
42. Munday & Blane, 1961
43. Nera, 1925
44. Prosser, et al. 1950
45. Robin, et al. 1964
46. Shoemaker, et al. 1966
47. Smith, 1929
48. Sutton, unpublished
49. Templeton, 1964
50. Urist & Schjeide, 1960/1961
51. Williams, Unpublished
52. Wilson, 1939
53. Wright & Jones, 1957
54. Zarafonetis & Kalas, 1960
55. Verbiinskaya, 1944
56. Tucker, 1966
57. Stenroos & Bowman, 1968
58. Moberly, 1968a, b
59. Tercafs & Vassas, 1967
60. Clark, 1967
61. Bradshaw & Shoemaker, 1967
62. Bolten & Bjondal, 1992

TABLE 13
PACKED CELL VOLUME AND CERTAIN ORGANIC CONSTITUENTS OF BLOOD

SPECIES	PCV (%)	Hbg (gm%)	T.P. (gm%)	Glucose mg/dl	Urea (mg/dl)	Uric Acid (mg/dl)	Reference*
TESTUDINES							
Chelydra serpentina	25	5.9**	4.7	33	96	2	6,13,20, 23,35,42
Kinosternon subrubrum	23	5.6					20,35
Sternotherus odoratus	33	11.2	4.5				20,35
Sternotherus minor	35	9.9	4.0				39,79
Deirochelys reticularia	20	8.3	4.2				35,39,79
Chrysemys picta	23	11.2	4.4	76	37	2	35, 37, 57, 70,75,79
Clemmys guttata		4.5**					20,71
Emys orbicularis	24	6.8**	6.1	50			2,35,52,54, 74
Malaclemys terrapin		9.2					39
Kachuga smithii				78			97
Pseudemys dorbigni				78			97

SPECIES	PCV (%)	Hbg (gm%)	T. P. (gm%)	Glucose mg/dl	Urea (mg/dl)	Uric Acid (mg/dl)	Reference*
Pseudemys scripta	26	8.0	3.6	70	22	1	20,35,36, 39,44,45
Pseudemys floridana							82
Testudo kleinmanni	27	8.1	6.6	78			60
Testudo hermanni							38
Terrapene carolina	28	5.9**	4.5	36	30	2	3,4,20,35, 37,50
Gopherus polyphemus	30	3.5					35,79,102
Chelonia mydas **	30 35.2	6.6**	2.9 5.1	114 60	52 7	8 1.5	8,35,58,62, 79,102,105
Caretta caretta	32	4.7			45		12,32,35, 62,85,102
Dermochelys coriacea		3.8		70		4	12,30
Trionyx ferox							20,35
Lissemys punctata			5.3	46			97
Pelusios sp.			4.3				35
Chelodina longicollis			3.3	99			35
Phrynops geoffroanus							34
SQUAMATA (Sauria)							
Gekko gecko				93	4		20
Coleonyx variegatus				94	4		39,83

Species							
Hemidactylus spp	10.8						39,97
Anolis carolinensis	28	7.0**	4.1	54	7	8	20,51,67
Crotaphytus collaris		7.8		172			19
Ctenosaura acanthura	35	6.0**	6.8	192	2	4	43
Iguana iguana	30	7.1**	4.5	155	1	5	43,79,102
Phrynosoma cornutum		7.0**	4.4	191	2		19,93
Phrynosoma douglassii		7.7**					19
Phrynosoma modestum		9.1**					19
Sauromalus obesus	31	8.4**	4.9				26
Sceloporus clarkii		6.2**					19
Sceloporus graciosus		8.2**					19
Sceloporus jarrovi		6.1**					19
Sceloporus occidentalis		7.1**					19
Sceloporus poinsetti		7.5**					19
Sceloporus undulatus		7.2**					19,20
Uta stansburiana	35	6.5**					19,101
Cordylus cataphractus						1	20
Uromastix spp		4.6		120			97,104
Lacerta lacerta		9.0					2,74

121

SPECIES	PCV (%)	Hbg (gm%)	T. P. (gm%)	Glucose mg/dl	Urea (mg/dl)	Uric Acid (mg/dl)	Reference*
Lacerta viridis		4.6					65
Chamaeleo chameleon				173	3		20
Eumeces fasciatus		3.0		107			20
Eumeces obsoletus		9.4**		112			18,67,68
Anguis fragilis		11.3					2,29,74
Cnemidophorus sexlineatus				93			20
Cnemidophorus tigris		7.2**					19
Cnemidophorus sackii		8.7**					19
Tupinambis nigropunctatus		7.8			2		20,79
Tupinambis teguixin				104			72
Gerrhonotus (Elgaria) multicarinatus		7.2**	4.5				19,20
Ophisaurus ventralis	35	6.9	5.4		3		20
Heloderma horridum	30	8.0		45	1		94
Heloderma suspectum	26	8.1**	6.3	109			20,31,76
Varanus sp.	27		6.9	106	2		20,40,41, 60,97,103

SQUAMATA (Ophidia)

Boa constrictor	29		6.5	70			9,102
Lichanura				73	6	1	20,79
roseofusca							
Epicrates cenchria				93			9
Eryx johnii				25			97
Coluber constrictor	26		5.0	75	4	6	11,12,13, 20,48
Coluber constrictor	26		6.2	65			60
Coluber viridiflavus			4.5	52			78
Heterodon platyrhinos					5		20
Lampropeltis getulus	23		5.8	59	2	6	12,48,76, 77,79
Rhinocheilus lecontei				88	2		20
Xenodon merremii				55			47
Natrix cyclopion	37		6.5	65	5		20,39
Natrix natrix	33		4.3	57			69,80
Natrix tessellatus			6.2				59,60
Natrix rhombifera			5.5	30			20
Natrix sipedon	23		5.7	49	5		12,13,17, 20,22,23,48
Philodryas sp.							73
Thamnophis sirtalis	33	8.1	4.5	63	5		11,12,20, 22,79
Thamnophis elegans	25		4.0				20,22

123

SPECIES	PCV (%)	Hbg (gm%)	T.P. (gm%)	Glucose mg/dl	Urea (mg/dl)	Uric Acid (mg/dl)	Reference*
Thamnophis sauritus	30		4.4				20,33
Farancia abacura		7.5	4.9				20,39,79
Storeia dekayi		10.8	3.5				20,39
Micrurus nigrocinctus				107			9
Naja naja	28		4.4	29			12,13,79,97
Agkistrodon contortrix			5.2				20
Agkistrodon piscivorus	19		4.6	52	5	6	12,13,20, 23,48,76
Bothrops atrox				60			9,73
Crotalus atrox			5.2	60	1	2	20,23,64,79
Crotalus horridus	45	8.6	3.5	60	11	3	12,23,79
Crotalus ruber			5.2	70			9,12,13,20
Crotalus viridis			2.9	48	0	2	12,13,20
Vipera aspis		10.5	5.5	40	10	4	1,28,33
Vipera sp.				34			88,98
Typhlops sp.				84	1		20
CROCODILIA							
Alligator mississippiensis	20	7.1**	5.1	74	0	3	5,7,16,25, 46,102

Caiman sp.	26	8.6	5.9	20,24,79, 102
Crocodylus niloticus	35			60
Crocodylus acutus	26	9.0		9,24,102
			101	

*Numbers designate reference source listed below.
**Calculated from oxygen capacity measurement; values based upon oxygen capacity were given preference in tabulation
\#\#values obtained from juvenile wild turtles (Bolten, A. B. and Bjorndal, K. A. (1992) *J. Wildlife Dis.*, 28(3):407–413)

REFERENCES (see Frye, 1991 for specific literature citations)

1. Agid, et al. 1961a
2. Alder & Huber, 1923
3. Altland & Parker, 1955
4. Altland & Thompson, 1958
5. Andersen, 1961
6. Andreen-Svedberg, 1933
7. Austin, et al. 1927
8. Berkson, 1966
9. Britton & Kline, 1939
10. Carmichael & Petcher, 1945
11. Clark, 1953
12. Cohen, 1954
13. Cohen, 1955
14. Cohen & Strickler, 1958
15. Correa, et al. 1960
16. Coulson & Hernandez, 1964
17. Dantzler, 1967
18. Dawson, 1960
19. Dawson & Poulson, 1962
20. Dessauer, unpublished, 1952
21. Dessauer & Fox, 1959
22. Dessauer, et al. 1956
23. Deutsch & McShan, 1949
24. Dill & Edwards, 1931a, b
25. Dill & Edwards, 1935
26. Dill, et al. 1935
27. Dimaggio & Dessauer, 1963
28. Duguy, 1962

29. Duguy, 1963
30. Dunlap, 1955
31. Edwards & Dill, 1935
32. Fanard & Ranc, 1912
33. Fine, et al. 1954
34. Foglia, et al. 1955
35. Frair, unpublished, 1964
36. Frankel, et al. 1966
37. Gaumer & Goodnight, 1957
38. Gilles-Ballien & Schoffeniels, 1965
39. Goin & Jackson, 1965
40. Haggag, et al. 1965
41. Haggag, et al. 1966
42. Henderson, 1928
43. Hernandez & Coulson, 1951
44. Hirschfeld & Gordon, 1961
45. Hirschfeld & Gordon, 1965
46. Hopping, 1923
47. Houssay & Biasotti, 1933
48. Hutton, 1958
49. Hutton, 1960
50. Hutton & Goodnight, 1957
51. Hutton & Ortman, 1957
52. Issekutz & Vegh, 1928
53. Izard, et al. 1961
54. Kanungo, 1961
55. Kaplan, 1960b
56. Kaplan & Rueff, 1960
57. Karr & Lewis, 1916
58. Khalil, 1947
59. Khalil & Abdel-Messieh, 1962
60. Khalil & Abdel-Messieh, 1963
61. Korzhuev & Kruglova, 1957
62. Lewis, 1964
63. Lopes, 1955
64. Luck & Keeler, 1929
65. Lustig & Ernst, 1936
66. McCay, 1931
67. Miller & Wurster, 1956
68. Miller & Wurster, 1958
69. Munday & Blanc, 1961
70. Mussachia & Sievers, 1962
71. Payne & Burke, 1964
72. Penhos, et al. 1965
73. Prado, 1946a
74. Prosser, et al. 1950
75. Rapatz & Mussachia, 1957
76. Rapoport & Guest, 1941

77. Rhaney, 1948
78. Saviano & DeFrancisis, 1948
79. Seal, 1964
80. Seniow, 1963
81. Sheeler & Barber, 1965
82. Southworth & Redfield, 1925/1926
83. Sutton, unpublished (undated)
84. Steggerda & Essex, 1957
85. Tercafs, et al. 1963
86. Vars, 1934
87. Vladescu, 1964, 1965b
88. Vladescu, 1965a
89. Wagner, 1955
90. Wiley & Lewis, 1927
91. Wilson, 1939
92. Wilson, et al. 1960
93. Wolfe, 1939
94. Zarafonetis & Kalas, 1960
95. Verbiinskaya, 1944
96. Tucker, 1966
97. Zain-ul-Abedin & Qazi, 1965
98. Stenroos & Bowman, 1968
99. Marques & Kraemer, 1968
100. Rao & David, 1967
101. Hadley & Burns, 1967
102. Thorson, 1968
103. Menon, 1952
104. Khalil & Yanni, 1959
105. Bolten & Bjorndal, 1992

TABLE 14
SUMMARY OF REPTILIAN BLOOD CELL HISTOCHEMISTRY

BLOOD CELL TYPE	ERYTHRO-CYTE	EOSINO-PHIL	HETERO-PHIL	BASO-PHIL	MONO-CYTE	THROMBO-CYTE	LYMPHO-CYTE
ENYZYMES							
Acid Phosphatase	+	+	+	+ −	+	+	+ −
Alkaline Phosphatase	−	+	+ −	+ −	+	−	+ −
Beta Glucuronidase	−	+	+	+	+	ND	+
Esterase	−	+ −	+	+ −	ND	ND	ND
Peroxidase	+	+	+ −	−	+ −	−	−
Lactic Acid Dehydrogenase	+	ND	ND	ND	ND	ND	ND
POLYSACCHARIDES							
Periodic Acid-Schiff	+ −	+	+	+	+	+	+ −

Alcian Blue	ND	+	–	+	ND	ND	ND
Toluidine Blue	ND	–	+	–	+	–	–
Astrablau	ND	–	–	+	ND	ND	ND
LIPIDS							
Sudan Black B	–	+ –	+	–	+	–	–
Acidic Nile Blue Sulfite	ND	–	+	ND	ND	ND	ND
Neutral Sudan III	ND	–	–	ND	ND	ND	ND
NUCLEIC ACIDS							
Methyl-Green Pyronin	ND	+	+	+	ND	ND	ND
Acridine Orange	ND	+	+	+	ND	ND	ND
Feulgen Reagent	ND	ND	ND	+	ND	ND	ND
BASIC PROTEINS							
Arginine	ND	ND	ND	–	ND	ND	ND
Bierbrich scarlet	ND	ND	ND	–	ND	ND	ND

BLOOD CELL TYPE	ERYTHRO-CYTE	EOSINO-PHIL	HETERO-PHIL	BASO-PHIL	MONO-CYTE	THROMBO-CYTE	LYMPHO-CYTE
Ninhydrin	ND	1,4,6,8	ND	1,4,6,8	ND	ND	ND
REFERENCES	1–3,7	1,4,6,8	1,4–6,8	–	1,2,8	2,5,8	1,2,8

Table reproduced with the permission of Sypek and Borysenko, 1988

References (see Frye, 1991 for specific literature citations):

1. Caxton-Martins, 1977
2. Caxton-Martins & Nganwuchu, 1978
3. Dessauer, 1970
4. Desser, et al. 1978
5. Desser & Weller, 1979a
6. Efrati, et al. 1970
7. Gerzeli, 1954
8. Pienaar, 1962

TABLE 15
SUMMARY OF REPTILIAN GRANULOCYTES AND MONOCYTES

BLOOD CELL TYPE	SIZE IN MICRONS	SHAPE OF NUCLEUS	BENZIDINE PEROXIDASE			METHYL GREEN PYRONIN	ACID FUCHSIN	HP-IGHT	ANILINE CRYSTAL VIOLET	P.A.S. MCDONALD	PAS DIGESTION	PHOSPHO-LIPIDS SUDAN BLACK	REFERENCES
			NEUTRAL	ALKALINE	ACID RED								
EOSINO-PHIL	9–20	round to oval	+	+	+	orange red	blue blk	+	+	−	+	+	1–3, 5–7, 9

Cell	Size	Shape								Cytoplasm	Granules					Refs
HETERO-PHIL	10–23	oval fusiform	+	–	–					muddy brown or orange-pink	blue blk	+	+	+	?	2–3, 5,8–9
BASO-PHIL	7–20	Oval	ND	ND	+					deep blue, metachromatic	ND	ND	–	–	+	2–3, 7,9
														+	–	
MONO-CYTE	8–20	vary	ND	ND	+					light blue-grey or azure	ND	ND	–	+	+	+	1,3, 5–7,9

Table modified and reproduced with the permission of Sypek and Borysenko, 1988.

References for TABLE 15 (see Frye, 1991 for literature citations):

1. Borysenko, 1976b
2. Desser & Weller, 1979b
3. Efrati, et al. 1970
4. Frye, 1981
5. Kelenyi & Nemeth, 1969
6. Mead & Borysenko, 1984a
7. Pienaar, 1962
8. Ryerson, 1943
9. Saint Girons, 1970

CHAPTER 4

CLINICAL METHODS

OBTAINING AN ADEQUATE HISTORY

I have developed several protocols to aid in the gathering of relevent information when dealing with reptile patients and their diseases. Three of these forms are reproduced at the end of this text for your convenience. The first is used in clinical situations and is filled out by each reptile-owning client and becomes part of the permanent record for each animal. The second is employed when investigating colony and/or multi-animal collection situations. The third is a pathology submission form that accompanies specimens submitted for histopathological examination and evaluation. If you wish, feel free to modify them for your own use.

PHYSICAL RESTRAINT AND TRANSPORT

Usually the safest way to handle captive reptiles is by means of transfer boxes or bags into which the animals often retreat voluntarily. Ideally, these animals should be handled only when absolutely necessary; the use of gloves, tongs, and nooses creates a potential problem of unintentional injury from the handler's inability to control the amount of pressure on the animals. Venomous snakes and lizards pose other problems, as do very aggressive lizards, crocodilians, large turtles, and some nonvenomous snakes. When necessary, a snake hook or long-handled net can be employed to handle snakes that, because of their teeth, venom, or overt aggressiveness, require remote manipulation. Sometimes placing a soft towel or large opaque cloth over an aggressive reptile makes it possible to manually restrain and handle it. Using a snake hook or encouraging venomous or very aggressive reptiles to enter transfer or squeeze cages is advised so that visual inspection, blood samples, or other procedures can be performed without injury to either the animal or its handler. If tongs must be used, jaw pressure only sufficient to hold the animal should be applied because these instruments can injure reptiles when used without care.

Because a reptile has but a single occipital condyle supporting its skull upon its cranial cervical spine, rough handling can cause a dislocated or fractured neck with attendant spinal cord injury. For this reason, the recommended technique for handling these animals (particularly snakes) is to support the head and neck gently in such a fashion that the balance of the body's weight is not borne by these relatively delicate structures. This is especially true when handling large heavy-bodied boas, pythons and anacondas which may weigh well over 125 kg (ca 275 lb), and some adult vipers and pit vipers that can weigh more than 8–10 kg. Often it is easier to coax one of these large snakes into a hiding box or bag held open with a long-handled snake hook. Once the snake enters the sack, the sack is closed and the open end secured with stout cordage, being certain to keep the sack well away from your body while doing so. Dangerous snakes often can be induced into, and restrained by, squeeze boxes that are attached to the back of their cage. Portable squeeze boxes also are useful. Moreover, the transparent plastic sheet that is used to compress the snake into the lowermost portion of the box is fitted with a handle and can be used separately as a shield to help crowd an aggressive animal into a corner of its cage, thus allowing safe access to the cage interior.

Many lizards and a few snakes can autotomize their tails as a defense against predators. Other snakes may suffer degloving injury to the caudal appendage if they are picked up by their tails. These characteristics can lead to some nasty clinical embarrassments if these animals are handled incorrectly. Although the lost portion of the tail will regenerate in lizards, the newly grown appendage will be less colorful and/or shorter than the original.

Many turtles and tortoises can deliver severe bites to unwary handlers, particularly during procedures that place the hands or fingers within the striking range of the sharp jaws of these animals. Simply covering the head, neck, and forelimbs with a cloth towel or sack and holding it in place with tape or elastic bands often is sufficient to prevent injury to the handler. If it is necessary to prevent an unanesthetized turtle or tortoise from walking during a procedure, the animal can be kept on an appropriate broad-based upturned cooking pot, flower pot, brick, or similar object. This will keep the chelonian's limbs from touching the substrate and effectively keep it from walking. Similarly, these animals can be kept in dorsal recumbency by inverting them and placing cloth, plastic foam, or sandbag bolsters inserted on either side of the carapace. These techniques are particularly useful during shell and horny mouthpart repairs. Alternatively, its legs can be confined within the shell by wrapping them and the overlying carapace and plastron with elastic bandage. Once the legs are immobilized in this manner, the animal can be placed on a pedestal from which it cannot escape by moving its head, neck, or legs.

Occasionally, the need arises to restrain a turtle or tortoise while its head is fully withdrawn from beneath its overlying shell. This maneuver can best be accomplished by using straight ovoid delivery forceps. The cervical spine of most chelonians is carried in a sigmoid curve which allows for withdrawal of the head and neck beneath the shell. In the cryptodiran chelonians, the sigmoid curve is vertically curved; in the pleurodiran, or side-neck turtles, it is laterally curved and the head is carried to one side of the midline, just beneath the cranial overhang of the carapace. In either case, the elongated neck can be extended easily by applying steady gentle traction by grasping the head with the forceps and applying only enough tension to overcome the turtle's efforts to keep its head beneath the shell. The main force of the forceps is applied away from the shell and not on the head itself. The holes of the forceps' jaws are placed so that the metallic rims do not touch the turtle's eyes.

Venomous or very active snakes can be put into clear, rigid-walled plastic tubes into which strategically placed holes or slots have been drilled. These tubes are convenient for restraint during injections and radiographic examinations. The ends of the tubes are fitted with secure caps or plug-like stoppers. When daily treatment is required, the snake can be safely kept in a tube for a few days, as long as strict attention is paid to the snake's fluid intake and excretory functions. These plastic tubes are not generally recommended for many of the elapid snakes (cobras, kraits, mambas, etc.) because these limber species may be able to turn around and bite the handler. When a snake hook must be used to pin down or control a venomous or aggressive nonvenomous snake, a suitable soft and resilient padded surface is useful to help restrain the animal and to prevent trauma. A piece of rubberized upholstery material or foam rubber serves this purpose very well. Nooses or cable "come-alongs" can be used, but can be dangerous to both the animal and the handler if the quick-release mechanism fails to disengage when freed.

Where chemical restraint is necessary, a subanesthetic dose of one of the rapid-acting, short duration injectable anesthetic agents can be useful. The use of these agents will be discussed later in this monograph (see CHEMICAL RESTRAINT/ANESTHESIA).

An old method for restraint was the use of hypothermia. A reptile would be placed into a refrigerator or freezer just long enough to induce a state of torpor. There are several serious disadvantages to this practice: (1) there is no evidence that lowering the body temperature of a reptile to the point where it can no longer respond to external stimuli necessarily abolishes the perception of pain; (2) the creature may suddenly awaken as it warms; if the animal is a hazardous species, there is the attendant danger to the handler(s); (3) the animal may die if it is left in the cold too long; (4) varying degrees of stress and immunodeficiency can be induced by hypothermia because vital immunoglobulin synthesis is temperature-dependent; too often, the sequel to a period of sudden hypothermia is respiratory infection. With the number of safe and effective chemical restraint agents available, the use of hypothermia for short-term restraint should be abandoned; however, profound hypothermia can be employed to induce death. Some reptiles, particularly montane lizards, can withstand profound cold temperatures for several hours of even days without apparent harm.

Crocodilians may experience hypoglycemia when excited or handled roughly. Although this hypoglycemia can be treated with oral or parenteral glucose therapy, it is better to avoid the stress altogether by applying only sufficient restraint or force to accomplish a particular procedure.

THE USE OF INDUCED VAGO-VAGAL RESPONSE FOR SHORT-TERM RESTRAINT

Crocodilians, most large lizards, and some chelonains can be immobilized for short periods by the application of gentle inward digital pressure upon their eyes for a few moments. Usually the effect of this vago-vagal response is observed after about 20–30 seconds. The depression of the eyes induces a brief drop in heart rate and blood pressure. An animal so treated will remain torpid for a few minutes without ill effect. This technique is particularly useful for restraint during radiography or other painless procedures; it is not applicable for snakes and some chelonians. Loud noises or other significant external stimuli abolish this response, but the pressure on the closed eyes can be repeated, as necessary.

CHEMICAL RESTRAINT/ANESTHESIA

A wide variety of chemical agents are available for sedating and anesthetizing reptiles. Because of their wide margin of safety, effectiveness, chemical stability under a broad range of temperatures, and availability, I will stress the use of the dissociative psychotropic agents ketamine HCl (Ketaset, Ketalar, Ketanest, Ketaject), at a dose of 20–50 mg/kg; teletamine-zolazepam (Telazol), at 10 mg/kg; and alfadolone acetate-alfaxalone acetate (Saffan), at an intravenous dosage of 6–9 mg/kg of the combined agent; they are highly effective in most reptiles and generally have a wide margin of safety. These potent agents can be injected intravenously or intramuscularly and when injected by the former route, induce sedation or anesthesia very rapidly, depending upon the dose. Arousal from surgical anesthesia usually is rapid and, if necessary, can be enhanced by intravenous injection of small volumes of diuretic agents and physiological fluids. Saffan should not be employed in patients who have been treated with dimethylsulfoxide (DMSO) because this agent can potentiate the anesthetic effects of aldolone-alfaxolone acetate. Barbiturates and other agents can be used, but with far less safety and consistency.

Inhalant anesthesia with volatile anesthetic agents such as methoxyflurane, halothane, and isoflurane produce excellent results and rapid recovery, but their use is limited under some conditions by the cost of the closed-circuit gas anesthetic equipment, the ambient temperature (and thus, the partial pressure of the volatilized gas), and the necessity for trained technical personnel. Because many reptiles will consciously hold their breath for prolonged periods and can survive hypoxia by employing anaerobic respiration, the use of nitrous oxide-oxygen is advised before adding one of the volatile gas anesthetic agents. The nitrous oxide-oxygen mixture is tasteless and odorless and reptiles usually become narcotized smoothly once the isoflurane or other agent is added after a few minutes exposure to the nitrous oxide-oxygen.

PREANESTHETIC PARASYMPATHOLYTIC MEDICATION

Premedication with atropine at 0.01–0.02 mg/kg, or glycopyrrolate (Robinul-V) at a dosage of 10.0 *micro*grams/kg

(0.050 ml/kg) is appropriate to reduce serous and mucous secretion and bradycardia. Glycopyrrolate is preferable to atropine because it delivers consistent results and its action is not prolonged.

TRANQUILIZERS

Although some of the phenothiazine-derivative tranquilizers can be used in reptiles, often they are not necessary. Two useful agents are acepromazine maleate and diazepam (Valium) which reduce the amount of anesthetic necessary; also, they provide muscle relaxation which is desirable in many orthopedic surgical procedures.

Paralyzing agents such as succinylcholine chloride (Sucostrin), curare, or tubocurarine have been employed in reptiles but their margin of safety is narrow and, thus, they should be reserved for special situations and by those who have had extensive experience with them. When employed, succinylcholine chloride should be used at a dosage of 0.5–1.5 mg/kg; the lowest dosage rate is preferred, and equipment for providing positive-pressure respiration must be available to support the patient's oxygen intake.

LOCAL, LINE, AND BLOCK ANESTHESIA

Lidocaine and procaine are effective in abolishing pain in reptiles, but the need to physically restrain the patient usually obviates the rationale for their use except under unusual field circumstances. When used, these products are injected along the proposed line of incision, or into the regional nerve supply to the area. Lidocaine is preferred. The addition of epinephrine is contraindicated because of its propensity for inducing prolonged vascular impedance which could lead to iatrogenic necrosis of digits or other extremities.

EUTHANASIA

If a reptile is to be euthanatized, it can be injected with any of the proprietory lethal solutions. Generally, an intravenous injection is preferred because if the cadaver is to be dissected to obtain tissues for histopathological processing and evaluation, these chemical agents may induce artifacts in the parenchymatous tissues in contact with the solution. This is particularly true with the myocardium and coelomic membrane-covered tissues. As mentioned earlier, a reptile can be placed into a freezer for a short time, but if destined for necropsy and histopathology, it should not be actually frozen. Decapitation of alert animals should be discouraged; the animal should be anesthetized, and then decapitated because there is evidence that decapitation does not produce instantaneous loss of consciousness.

PHYSICAL EXAMINATION

Although a routine physical examination may not be indicated for every captive reptile, there are good reasons for encouraging preventative health care. For example, those species which hibernate (*brumate*) can benefit greatly by careful evaluation before they are placed into their autumnal sleep and immediately after they return to activity in the spring. By performing this examination, the presence of preexisting disease, particularly respiratory infections, can be diagnosed and treated aggressively. Also, the body weight of the animal should be determined and evaluated as to the advisability of subjecting the creature to the rigors of the prolonged (often 6 month) period of torpor. Underweight tortoises may not possess sufficient tissue stores to carry them through the entire period of hibernation (or brumation; a form of greatly lowered metabolic activity). The limbs are palpated for the presence of swollen joints and the entire animal is inspected for other swellings which may consist of abscesses, pyogranulomata, or tumors. Reptiles found to be affected by any significant disease condition should not be placed into hibernation, nor be permitted to enter it on their own volition unless and until the condition has been corrected. If this requires foregoing hibernation entirely, so be it. Prophylactic antibiotic treatment generally is not warranted in healthy animals being prepared for hibernation.

The post-hibernation examination is directed toward detecting the presence of respiratory infection, underweight, ophthalmic conditions, or other disorders. The animal is weighed, auscultated, palpated, and its oral cavity, oral mucous membranes and eyes are examined for the presence of abnormalities. Depending upon the size of the reptile being examined, the mouth may be opened with the fingers (many chelonians, some lizards and small crocodilians) or with a soft and flexible kitchen spatula, used by gently inserting the thin edge between the mandibles and maxillary (and premaxillary, where present) arcade. By lifting the handle of the spatula, the mouth is gently forced open. At this point, a visual inspection is made for the presence of parasites, broken teeth, infections or other inflammatory lesions, neoplasms, foreign bodies, and evidence of and reasons for malocclusion, etc.

Usually the urinary bladder can be palpated with the examiner's fingers inserted into the "pockets" just cranial to the hindlimbs. The tortoise is then gently rolled from side to side and the finger tips ballotte the bladder and its contents, as well as the oviducts. If either urinary bladder stones and/ or eggs are detected, a radiograph should be obtained to determine the size and shape of the calculus and/or shelled ova. Often, a warm bath immediately after removal of the animal from its hibernaculum will induce it to drink, defecate, and pass urates. The stools and urates may be quite inspissated because of the prolonged absorption of their moisture contents. As soon as they become available, feces should be examined microscopically for the presence of intestinal parasites.

Another rationale for encouraging yearly or periodic examinations is that many conditions, if observed and treated early in their course, can be resolved, whereas if permitted to exist for prolonged periods, they often become difficult to manage effectively. For example, many tumors and inflammatory lesions are relatively simple to extirpate when diagnosed and treated early. In some instances, urinary bladder stones, when small, can be dissolved by treating the animal with increased water intake and cranberry juice, or another dietary source of urinary acidification. In some cases, small stones can be removed entirely through the insertion of an appropriate instrument into the urethra and urinary bladder. Lastly, many traumatic and inflammatory lesions, particularly those involving the chelonian shell, can progress to serious consequences if left untreated for a prolonged period; when detected early and treated vigorously, most will heal with great rapidity; many of these same lesions can be very serious and difficult to resolve.

Another reason for periodic physical examination is to assess the fitness of particular reptiles for breeding. The production of sperm and ova, or embryos and fetuses, requires large amounts of energy and can be stressful for both sexes. Also, courtship behavior and the exaggerated territoriality that is often displayed are stressful. Thus, only those animals in good health and body condition should be selected for breeding. Any parasites found must be treated so that neither the adult nor resulting immature neonate reptiles are harmed by parasitic infestations which have direct life cycles and, thus, can be transmitted from reptile to reptile.

To this point, I have stressed those things that the veterinarian can do to prolong the life and health of a captive reptile. The owners of these animals should be encouraged to maintain accurate records on each animal they possess. The date when each was obtained, the source, any history of disease and/or treatment, dates and nature of each meal, dates and nature of all waste elimination and any history of reproduction, skin shedding, etc. should be recorded. In many instances, a personal visit to the collection or animal colony can be very rewarding. A general inspection and overview of the husbandry practices may lead to clues to why infectious diseases occur. The expense of such inspections is easily justified, particularly in those instances where the animals are rare, threatened, or endangered. Often the sources of foodstuffs are found to be substandard and can be directly responsible for disease outbreaks.

The application of most routine physical examination and diagnostic methods often are easily adapted to reptiles. There are exceptions, but these can be circumvented or replaced by other methods that will yield useful information.

The use of a rectal thermometer is limited in clinical reptile medicine because of the poikilothermic (or heterothermic) nature of this class of animals. Although some reptiles have been shown to mount a mild pyrexia in response to some pathogenic bacteria or their endotoxins, the magnitude of this febrile reaction is modest and is not likely to be detected with the clinical fever thermometers commonly in use.

Stethoscopy is useful in helping to evaluate the state of pulmonary function of some reptiles, particularly chelonians, crocodilians, the tuatara, and large lizards. It is less valuable in snakes. In order to employ a stethoscope to amplify the breath sounds of a scaly or plated reptile, some means must be used to damp out the background sounds of the instrument's diaphragm contact with the animal's irregular surfaces. This can most conveniently be accomplished by applying a piece of moist cotton towel against the patient's skin and then placing the stethoscope's diaphragm directly against the cloth (Frye & Himsel, 1988). By using this method, the breath sounds will be transmitted through the dampened cloth and will eliminate the unwanted sounds of the skin scraping against the stethoscope. Heart sounds are only rarely heard with routine stethoscopy but can be detected with electronically amplified instruments.

Electrocardiography can be applied to reptiles as it is to higher vertebrates. However, there is little published material describing myocardial conduction abnormalities with which to compare clinical cases. When the patient is legless, one merely places the needle electrodes where limbs would normally be located; RL and LL on either side of the cloacal vent area; RA and LA midway down the cervical region. In snakes and some lizards, a three-lead esophageal EKG probe made from a rubber or plastic urethral catheter can be used to very good effect; this device obviates the need for placing needle electrodes and has been employed at the Veterinary Medical Teaching Hospital, University of California, Davis for several years.

Conventional electrocardiography is a useful modality for investigating the characteristic electrical activity of the myocardial contraction and the innate conduction system; however, the miniscule size of many reptiles limits the use of electrocardiography even when a small-diameter esophageal catheter fitted with three or more isolated electrodes is employed. The Doppler ultrasonic echocardiographic flow detector offers a relatively new, non-invasive, moderately priced, highly sensitive, accurate and cost-effective alternative means for clinically evaluating intracardiac and intravascular sounds even in very small patients.

Echocardiography generally is used to detect the sound of blood flowing over and between the heart valves. In order to maintain a sound-transmitting medium between the surface of the patient and the surface of the transducer head, a layer of water-soluble gel, such as Aquasonic 100[(R)] ultrasound transmission gel (Parker Laboratories, Inc., Orange, NJ 07050 USA) or any other accoustic coupling gel is used. A product such as K-Y Lubricating Jelly (Johnson & Johnson Products, Inc., New Brunswick, NJ 08903 USA) has several advantages; it is readily available, nonirritating, inexpensive and yields a high quality signal that is equal to the more expensive products sold for clinical optical ultrasonography. The patient is restrained gently either in dorsal recumbancy or held by the operator with one hand as the detector's flat or slightly concave head (filled with water-soluble gel) is brought into contact with the patient's skin surface. Once the detector head has been brought into contact, the pushbutton switch on the handpiece is depressed and the sounds that are detected are heard on a small solid-state amplifier. In turn, these signals can be fed into a conventional audio amplification sytem so that the detected sounds can be heard by an unlimited number of people. Each Doppler detector is equipped with a potentiometer to adjust the loudness of the amplified signals heard through the speaker. An optional interface device is available from the manufacturer which permits the Doppler to be coupled to a conventional paper-strip electrocardiograph, thus producing a hard copy tracing.

When used in chelonians, the detector may be applied in one of two fashions: (1) the transducer is placed directly on the plastral surface immediately over the region of the single large ventricle; (2) when necessary, the patient contact surface of the transducer is applied to the soft tissues covering the region between the medial aspect of one forelimb and the neck. This places the detector directly over the location of the cranial cardiac structures and heart base, twin aortic arches, the brachiocephalic and carotid arteries, and jugular veins where they empty into the anterior vena cava. In both instances, a layer of water-soluble gel is used between the detector and the surface of the patient. The low velocity blood flowing within the paired dorsal occipital and vertebral sinuses can be detected as a soft "whooshing" sibilance when the Doppler detector is placed perpendicular to the longitudinal axis of the outstretched neck of turtles and tortoises.

For lizards, the detector is applied to a site on the midline, just cranial to the forelimbs; this placement generally is suitable for crocodilians also. The ventricular apical beat of snakes often can be seen when the animal is viewed in incident illumination; if the heart beat is not immediately visible, the gel-covered detector can be applied to the ventral midline commencing about 15% down the length of the snake and moved caudally until the sounds of the heart beat and blood flowing over and through the heart valves are heard.

Distinct differences in sound quality are easily discerned between chamber filling, ejection, and individual valvular and vascular structures. Blood flow in arteries is pulsatile and yields audio signals with a relatively high pitch; venous blood flow is of a lower frequency and is more constant, with a characteristic "swishing" sound. A signal generated at the site of a cardiovascular lesion or dysfunction has a different tone and amplitude, tending to increase or decrease depending upon the position of the detecting instrument in relation to the lesion. These lesions can be constrictions, such as valvular stenoses, mural thrombi, or other conditions which narrow the lumen of the valve or vessel. If a vessel is completely obstructed, the blood flow signal will be lost entirely as the Doppler is moved over the site of obstruction. In pregnant or gravid lizards, the heart may be shifted slightly cranial to its normal position which is approximately between the forelimbs. This change in position is induced by the presence of the fetuses or ova which can occupy a substantial volume and often displace the liver, stomach, lungs and heart to a more cranial location. The amount of pressure and the angle of the instrument affect the quality of the audio signal. The proper technique can be mastered quickly by listening to one's own heart, brachial, radial, digital, or carotid arteries.

After using the Doppler unit, remove the water-soluble gel from the surfaces of the patient and transducer head with cleansing tissue or a dampened sponge.

Two commercially available Doppler units* fitted with 2.25 MHz and 8 MHz crystal transducers have proven to be particularly useful in my practice. Table 1 contains the technical specifications for each of these instruments. These devices have detected abnormal cardiovascular sounds of loud atrioventricular and aortic valve murmurs arising from low-viscosity (anemic) ejection brûits, loud adventitious burbling of blood as it passes over knobby heart valves caused by chronic vegetative endocarditis, and a high-pitched murmur arising from congenital unilateral aortic stenosis. Each of these cases was confirmed histopathologically. Although I have seen only a single case of large-vessel aneurysm in a reptile, this technology should be capable of detecting the fremitus created in even deeply imbedded vascular aneurysmal lesions, thus making their antemortem diagnosis possible. Echocardiology may be useful in monitoring the

*Ultrascope Obstetrical Doppler, Model 2, 2.25 MHz; and Ultrascope Doppler Arterial and Venous Blood Flow Detector, Model 8, 8 MHz; EMS Predicts, Inc. 1130 8th St., Kirkland, WA 98033 USA; Telephone 1-206-827-5996; 1-800-926-9622.

The Model 2 has an external diameter of approximately 1.0 cm; Model 8 has an external diameter of approximately 0.5 cm and was designed specifically for detecting blood flow in small superficial vessels. Mention of any product is not necessarily an endorsement by the author.

embryonic viability of avian and reptilian embryos as they develop within their eggshells after conventional candling is no longer productive. Another use for audio Doppler ultrasonic echocardiography is the monitoring of intracoelomic fetal heartbeats in those species which retain the products of conception until the end of fetal development. This includes many snake species, especially boas, and some lizards, such as prehensile-tailed skinks. In larger reptiles, this equipment is useful for locating large vascular structures beneath thick and unyielding bony carapacial and plastral plates.

Percussion hammers are useful in eliciting neuromuscular reflexes in large reptiles and for percussing the lungfields. Smaller lizards and crocodilians can be induced to respond to tendon taps by using the finger rings of various size forceps or similar metallic objects to percuss the patellar, Achilles, or other tendons.

Direct and indirect ophthalmoscopy is employed in an identical fashion to that utilized in higher vertebrates. The use of homatropine or similar mydriatic agents to dilate the iris diaphragm is *in*effective in reptiles because of the presence of skeletal rather than smooth muscle fibers in the reptilian eye. In this case, apply d-tubocurarine topically to dilate the pupils. Induced mydriasis is particularly valuable when examining reptiles with a slit-like eliptical pupil shape, but then again, these pupils are only found in crocodilians, some lizards and some snakes; some of these lizards (the geckos) lack moveable eyelids and have spectacle-like shields covering their corneae which inhibit the absorption of ophthalmic drops into the interior of the eye where these agents produce paralysis of the skeletal muscle fibers.

Clinical hematology and physiological chemistry are particularly useful as adjuncts to a thorough physical examination. Screening tests utilizing chemical-impregnated paper or plastic strips are useful in assessing renal, hepatic and pancreatic functions. Suspicious findings are confirmed by clinical chemistry procedures.

Fine-needle biopsy of suspicious lesions should be employed to arrive at definitive diagnoses of such abnormalities. Of course, the skin of the reptilian patient must be scrubbed and prepared for the insertion of the sterile biopsy needle just as with a higher vertebrate.

A variety of rubber-like plastic kitchen spatulas are very useful as wedges with which the mouths of many snakes and lizards may be opened without inducing trauma. These devices are inexpensive, and can be easily cleaned and disinfected between uses.

FLUID REPLACEMENT AND MAINTENANCE THERAPY

Generally, fluids in the form of physiological saline, Ringer's or lactated Ringer's, dextrose-saline, etc. are administered at a rate of 15–25 ml/kg/24 hours. Unless the reptilian patient is critically dehydrated, intracoelomic and/or subcutaneous routes are employed, depending upon the volume that must be administered. If rapid expansion of the plasma volume is indicated, a "butterfly" infant scalp vein infusion set can be used to infuse sterile physiologic fluid into an appropriate vein such as the jugular, lateral sinus, postoccipital sinus, or ventral caudal vein. More critical cases can be treated via intravenous, intraosseous (intramedullary), or even intracardiac catheterization (Mader, personal communication). Intraosseous infusion is accomplished most practically in crocodilians, larger lizards, and some chelonians. After appropriate integumentary cleansing, a spinal or other stilette-equipped needle is inserted into the marrow cavity of the femur or humerus, via the trochanteric fossa or through the proximal (scapular) end of the humerus, respectively; in chelonians, the diploe-like carapace is pierced, the needle is advanced into the soft cancellous bone, and the fluid is injected. If these routes are employed, usual aseptic techniques and pericatheter care and antibiotic application are mandatory to help avoid dissemination of iatrogenic infection. A topical antibiotic ointment containing neomycin, bacitracin and/or polymyxin is used to surround the catheter-skin junction. The site is covered with a sterile dressing and is attended at least once daily as long as the catheter is inserted. Indwelling intravenous catheters can be left in situ for several days if necessary as long as they remain patent and free-flowing and sepsis is avoided. These indwelling devices should be flushed with dilute lithium heparin solution twice daily to inhibit intraluminal coagulation or thrombus formation.

BLOOD TRANSFUSION

The use of homologous, or even heterologous, blood transfusion has been employed in clinical reptile practice, much as it has been in avian medicine. The major problem with blood transfusion used to accomplish blood volume expansion has been the dearth of suitable blood donors. Whenever possible, a donor of at least the same genus of the patient requiring blood should be used. In emergency situations, a single heterologous transfusion can be used, but only with the owner's informed consent. If subsequent heterologous transfusions are to given, the blood must be cross-matched before it is infused. Anecdotal cases of avian-reptile transfusion have been described, but insufficient data are available to determine the useful lifespan of such cross-phylogenetic transfusions, or their long-term effects.

The injection sites for blood transfusion are the same as those employed for physiological fluid therapy. The use of the coelomic cavity for administering whole blood is not recommended.

OBTAINING DIAGNOSTIC MATERIAL FROM THE RESPIRATORY TRACT

Many of the techniques employed in small companion animal clinical veterinary medicine are entirely applicable to reptilian patients. These techniques include tracheal sampling, transtracheal lavage, and choanal slit microbiological and cytological swabbing. Tiny microswabs make these methods practical in even very small reptiles. One of the simplest methods for assessing the presence of inflammatory cells or parasites and/or their ova or larvae is to inert a saline-moistened cotton bud-tipped applicator into the laryngeal orifice. The specimen is then rolled gently onto a clean glass microscopic slide, air-dried, and stained with New Methylene Blue, Gram's, or any of several brands of Wright's or Giemsa stain, or even merthiolate, coverslipped, and examined microscopically. If heterophil granulocytes are found in large numbers, they are suggestive of microbial infection.

Suspected cases of infection should be submitted for microbiological culture and sensitivity testing. Lactol-phenol/cotton blue stain can be used to help identify fungal elements in the sputum. If fungi are suspected, a sterile swab can be used to inoculate a rapid fungal detection medium which is then incubated at room temperature.

Trematode helminths can be removed from the upper respiratory tract and pharynx with a dry cotton-tipped applicator stick. Identification can be made from acid-formalin-alcohol (AFA)-fixed specimens or from fresh material that has been immersed in Hoyer's medium and mounted beneath a coverslip.

OBTAINING DIAGNOSTIC MATERIAL FROM THE CAUDAL ALIMENTARY TRACT

If a small stool specimen is required from an animal who has not defecated, an adequate sample often can be obtained by employing a smooth-edged plastic spoon-like device that is inserted into the cloacal vent. Failing this, a small volume of physiologic fluid or tap water can be introduced into the cloacal vault afterwhich the caudal portion of the animal's body is agitated to flush feces from the colonic or rectal wall. The fluid is then collected and processed routinely to produce a useful fecal specimen. Mayer's hematoxylin, New Methylene Blue, Lugol's iodine, or merthiolate can be added to stain ova, parasitic protozoa, etc. and, thus, make them easier to identify microscopically.

ELECTROPHYSICAL CHARACTERISTICS OF TWO ULTRASONIC DOPPLERS*
(Maximum Values of Intensity and Ultrasonic Power in Water)

MODEL	INTENSITY		TRANSMIT APERTURE DIMENSION	NOMINAL ULTRASONIC TRANSMIT FOCAL LENGTH (cm)	-6db BEAM POWER (Mv)	CROSS SECTIONAL AREA
2	[I]SPTA (mW/cm^2)	13.5	1.27 cm half circle	0.8	1.64	0.150
2.25 MHz	[I]SPPA (W/cm^2)	0.0135	1.27 cm half circle	0.8	1.64	0.150
	[I]M (W/cm^2)	0.0135	1.27 cm half circle	0.8	1.64	——
	[I]SATA (mW/cm^2)	2.6				
8	[I]SPTA (mW/cm^2)	6.02	1.27 cm half circle	0.6	1.10	0.261
8.0 MHz	[I]SPPA (W/cm^2)	0.006	1.27 cm half circle	0.6	1.10	0.261
	[I]M (W/cm^2)	0.006	1.27 cm half circle	0.6	1.10	——
	[I]SATA (mW/cm^2)	1.74				

Legend:
[I]SPTA = Spatial Peak Temporal Average Intensity
[I]SPPA = Spatial Peak Pulse Average Intensity
[I]M = Maximum Intensity
[I]SATA 3 Spatial Average Transmission Aperture Intensity (at transducer face): Model 2 = 2.6 mW/cm^2; Model 8 = 1.74 mW/cm^2 These results are less than the greatest known pre-enactment value of 20 mW/cm^2.
*Data courtesy of EMS Products Inc.

TABLE 16
CHEMICAL RESTRAINT AND ANESTHETIC AGENTS

DRUG	DOSAGE mg/kg	ROUTE	COMMENTS/PRECAUTIONS
SUCCINYLCHOLINE CHLORIDE (Sucostrin[R] and Anectine[R] Burroughs Wellcome)	0.5–1.5	IM	Narrow margin of safety; Artificial respiration may be required
GALLAMINE TRIETHIODIDE (Flaxedil[R] Abbott, Boehringer)	1.0 to 1.25	IM	Reverse with 0.25 mg of neostigmine
TUBOCURARINE (Abbott)	1.8 (pythons) 6.0 (Australian colubrid snakes)	IM	Artificial respiration may be required
PENTOBARBITAL SODIUM (Nembutal[R] Abbott; Sagatal[R] May & Baker Pentobarbital[R] Borhringer)	7.7–20 (crocodilians) 15–30.0 (snakes) 10–16 (chelonians) 11–22 (iguanas)	IM/IV IM/IC IM/IC IM/IC	Narrow margin of safety
THIOPENTAL SODIUM (Pentothal[R] Abbott; Intraval[R] May & Baker)	15–30	IM/IV/I/C	Narrow margin of safety
THIAMYLAL SODIUM (Surital[R] Parke-Davis)	15–30	IV	Dilute to 2.0%

Drug	Dose	Route	Notes
METHOHEXITAL SODIUM (Brevital[R] Eli Lilly)	5–20	IV	Highly variable results
KETAMINE HCL (Ketaset[R] Bristol); (Ketalar[R], Vetalar[R], Ketaject[R], Ketanest[R] Parke-Davis)	20–60	IM/IV	Dilute with saline if delivered IV
TELETAMINE HCL/ZOLAZEPAM (Telazol[R] A. H. Robins)	10–30	IM/IV	Do not use in association with ivermectin within 10 days
XYLAZINE (Rompun[R])	0.10–1.25	IM/IV	
FENTANYL-DROPERIDOL (Innovar-Vet[R] Pitman-Moore); (Sublimaze[R] Janssen) ml/kg	0.20 ml/kg	IM	Highly variable results; not recommended
TRICAINE METHANE-SULPHONATE (MS 222) (Finquel[R] Sandoz)	15–200 70–110 crocodilians	IM	Used mostly in fish & amphibians Prolonged anesthesia

DRUG	DOSAGE mg/kg	ROUTE	COMMENTS/PRECAUTIONS
TRIBROMETHANOL-AMYLENE HYDRATE (Avertin[R] Bayer, Squibb)	250 tribromo methanol, plus 125 mg amylene hydrate; tortoise dose	IC	Can also be administered by intracloacal instillation at 0.4 ml/kg of the mixture. DO NOT USE IN DEBILITATED ANIMALS
ETORPHINE HCL AND DIPRENORPHINE HCL (M-99[R] Lemmon); (M 50–50[R] Lemmon)	0.15–5.0 0.5–20 crocodilians Double the dose of etorphine injected for reversal	IM	EXTREME CAUTION MUST BE TAKEN TO AVOID ACCIDENTAL INJECTION INTO HUMANS; DIPRENORPHINE MUST BE IMMEDIATELY AVAILABLE AS ANTIDOTE
OXYMORPHONE (P/M Oxymorphone[R] HCl Pitman-Moore; Numorphone[R] DuPont & Endo)	0.025–0.10 0.5–1.5 snakes	IV IM	DO NOT USE IN PATIENTS WITH HEPATIC OR RENAL INSUFFICIENCY REVERSE WITH NALOXONE
ALPHAXALONE-ALPHADOLONE ACETATE (Saffan[R] Glaxo)	9.0 9.0–18.0 (0.75–1.5 ml)	IV IM	DO NOT USE WITHIN 10 DAYS OF DMSO TREATMENT

Drug	Dosage	Route	Notes
METHOXYFLURANE (Metofane[R] Pitman-Moore)	INDUCTION @ 3–4% MAINTAIN @1.5–2.0%		Human health hazard; avoid exposure to gas mixture
HALOTHANE (Fluothane[R] Ayerst)	INDUCTION @ 3–4% MAINTAIN @1.5–2.0%		Human health hazard; avoid exposure to gas mixture
ISOFLURANE (AERrane[R] Anaquest/BOC)	INDUCTION @3–4% MAINTAIN @1.5–3.0%		Avoid unnecessary exposure
NITROUS OXIDE	INDUCTION @1:1–1:2 $NO_2:O_2$ ADDED TO VOLATILE GAS		Potential for human abuse
TRANQUILIZERS (Acepromazine maleate[R] Ayerst)	0.1–0.5 mg/kg	IM	REDUCE DOSAGE OF INJECTABLE ANESTHETIC(S)
Chlorpromazine hydrochloride (Thorazine[R] Smith-Kline; Megaphen[R] Bayer);	0.1–0.5 mg/kg	IM	REDUCE DOSAGE OF INJECTABLE ANESTHETIC(S)
Promazine (Sparine[R] Wyeth)	0.1–0.5 mg/kg	IM	REDUCE DOSAGE OF INJECTABLE ANESTHETIC(S)

CHAPTER 5

SOME PRACTICAL SURGICAL AND NON-SURGICAL PROCEDURES

Most of the surgical procedures performed upon small companion pet animals are appropriate in captive reptiles. Exploratory celiotomy, gastrointestinal procedures such as gastrotomy and enterotomy, intestinal resection and anastomosis, gastro-, colo-, and urocystopexy, pneumonectomy, partial hepatic resection, partial pancreatectomy, splenectomy, nephrectomy, salpingotomy, hysterectomy, ovariectomy, orchiectomy, vasectomy, venom adenectomy, open-reduction fracture repair, chelonian shell repair, ocular enucleation, limb amputation, spinal neurosurgery, and restorative repair of severe ratbite trauma are procedures that have been described in the expanding literature. All of these surgical procedures are well within the capability of today's veterinary surgeons. While the anatomy and, thus, surgical approaches differ widely between many of these animals, they do not pose insurmountable obstacles to innovative surgeons.

The most common surgical problems seen in practice tend to be related to (1) the popularity of any particular species (currently, the common green iguana is the most popular pet reptile), (2) whether it is a natural hibernator or not,

(3) the particular season of the year, and (4) improper nutrition.

ANESTHESIA

The choice of anesthesia employed often is dictated by the nature of the reptilian patient and/or its immediate pre-operative condition. Whenever possible, use volatile agents, particularly isoflurane, delivered via a closed-circuit system. Other agents that have been used with excellent results are alfoxolone acetate-aldolone acetate (Saffan[R]), ketamine HCl, teletamine HCl-zolazopam (Telazol[R]), etc. In some instances, a local, line, or field block with infiltrated 1–2% lidocaine is indicated. Local anesthesia is particularly useful in reducing prolapses of the cloacal membrane, rectum, colon, oviduct, penis (or hemipenis) and during the immediate postoperative period of healing because it greatly or completely abolishes tenesmus and, thus, helps preserve the integrity of the organ in its restored position.

FRACTURES

Because of improper nutrition and lack of suitable caging, longbone and spinal fractures are common. These fractures sometimes involve grossly osteopenic bones and, as a result, applying internal fixation in the form of pins, rods or plates is not suitable; therefore, external coaptation splintage must be used. Whenever applied for immobilization of a limb, make certain that the splint is well padded with cast padding and held in place firmly so that wrinkles are avoided and that pressure is not applied to regional vascular structures. In the properly fed, mature animal, intramedullary pinning or bone plating often is the treatment of choice.

GASTROTOMY AND ENTEROTOMY

Gastrotomy for the removal of ingested foreign bodies, gastroliths, severe gastric ulceration, and gastric neoplasms is routine since reptiles are monogastric; incision and closure in these creatures are identical to when operating upon mammals. Partial enterectomy for successful reduction of gastroduodenal and duodenojejunal intussusception, or mural neoplasms, is performed as on any of the higher vertebrates, except for snakes. The ophidian pancreas and biliary drainage systems differ because the pancreas—which usually forms a complex of the spleen and gallbladder—is substantially distant from the liver. The pancreas in snakes tends to be a firm pyramidal mass, usually containing a nonrandom distribution of islet tissue. Enterotomy into the *small* intestine is routine and is largely performed as it is in mammals. However, because many herbivorous reptiles employ hindgut fermentation in order to process cellulose and other nutritive fiber, the multiloculated and usually enlarged colon and cecum are particularly thin-walled and must be handled with exquisite care, using minimal instrumentation. I prefer using my fingers whenever possible to avoid having to immobilize these delicate organs.

PROLAPSES

Prolapse of the colon, rectum, urinary bladder, oviduct, and even a kidney has been recorded in reptiles. Often, when the colon or rectum are involved, the inciting cause is intestinal parasitism. Therefore, in order for the surgical repair to be successful, the underlying etiology of the condition must be corrected. Depending upon the nature of the prolapsed organ(s) and their condition, the structure is either replaced into its natural intracoelomic site or excised. Apply glycerine or concentrated sucrose solution to help reduce the induration. If necessary, make an episotomy-like relieving incision to facilitate replacement of a swollen viscus organ. Most colo-, entero-, and urocystopexies require open celiotomy to afford adequate exposure. In lizards and snakes however, some of these procedures can be performed transcutaneously once the organ has been reduced manually. Insert a lubricated gloved finger of your non-dominant hand into the cloacal vent and use it to immobilize the segment of rectum or colon against the body wall. A glass or plastic test tube or plastic urethral catheter container can be used in lieu of your finger; however, being able to actually feel the passage of the needle is a distinct advantage because you can judge if the depth of each suture as it penetrates the intestinal wall is sufficient to hold the organ securely without tearing at the points of fixation. If the patient is too small to permit the insertion of a finger, use a cotton-tipped applicator stick or polypropylene urethral catheter. Place one or more sutures carried on a taper-point needle into, but not completely through, the wall of the gut or urinary bladder, using your finger or other obturator to help guide the placement of each suture tuck. Have an assistant tie the knots as they are placed by your dominant hand. Use only sufficient tension to hold the gut—or other prolapsed organ—to the muscular lateral or ventral body wall.

SALPINGOTOMY/CAESARIAN DELIVERY

Salpingotomy and/or caesarian delivery of the products of conception are commonly performed in oviparous reptiles, but much less so in ovoviviparous and viviparous species. These procedures often are necessary due to the collapse or fracture of calcareous eggshells whose sharp edges impinge upon the thin and delicate lining of the oviducts. Placing temporary or permanent stay sutures on either side of the proposed line of incision into the oviductal wall greatly aids in not only maintaining an open stoma, but also in closing the operative wound at the conclusion of surgery.

Place stay sutures in the urinary bladder *before* making the cystotomy incison. Once the bladder has been evacuated and flushed, these sutures greatly facilitate closure and, thus, reduce surgery time and effort.

ORBITAL ENUCLEATION

Enucleation of the orbital contents in most lizards, chelonians, and crocodilians differs little from the same surgery in mammals. However, because they lack movable eyelids, snakes and some lizards pose a problem in mobilizing sufficient skin to cover the operative defect. Sliding skin grafts, conventional Z-plasties, etc. usually do not yield enough skin to suture over the orbital wound. The liquid plastic antiseptic bandages such as New Skin[R] do, however, permit fibroplastic filling of the defect in a short time with satisfactory cosmetic appearance once the integument has regenerated over the fibrocollagenous connective tissue which fills the operative site.

INCISION AND REPAIR OF THE CHELONIAN SHELL

The two techniques that have been employed for entering the coelomic cavity of hard-shelled turtles, tortoises, and terrapins are (1) transplastral and (2) soft-tissue. In the latter, one or more incisions are placed in the region of the rear limb fossae; although this approach can be useful, it somewhat limits exposure to the intracoelomic viscera and offers only a small area through which large objects can be removed from the coelom. The transplastral technique which permits more generous observation, exploration, and instrumentation is described in detail.

Make incisions through the keratin-covered bony plastron of hard-shelled chelonians with rotary, oscillating, or high-speed turbine-powered orthopedic saws or drills with an appropriate cutting blade or bur. For most small-to medium-size chelonians weighing up to 10 kg, use a hand-held electric rotary drill fitted with a circular saw blade to enter the coelomic cavity. Because the shells of heavily buttressed tropical American, European, African, and Asian tortoises are significantly thicker than those of temperate North American species, small-diameter circular saw blades cannot fully penetrate the plastron; also, most high-speed turbine-powered burs have insufficient length or torque to cut all the way through this bone. Therefore, use a Stryker[R] (Stryker Corp.) or Richards oscillating saw fitted with a 10 cm blade (originally designed for necropsy examination of the spinal column and its contents). Create a 45° angled bevel on the cut surfaces with the greatest dimension nearest the outer surface. This bevel effectively holds the celiotomy bone flap in place while it is being secured at the end of the procedure.

To help determine the site for the plastral incision, make a survey radiograph to ascertain the position of the pelvic and brachial girdles and the size of the hole that will have to be created. The plastral opening must be large enough to permit the removal of any intact urinary calculi, intraoviductal ova or masses, and to admit the entrance of instruments, and/or the surgeon's hands. It is better to make the celiotomy hole slightly larger than necessary because it will be extremely difficult to enlarge it once the flap has been removed or to close a modified surgical wound later. Once the full thickness of the plastron has been incised, detach the bony flap from the rectus muscle with a periosteal elevator and place it in saline or Ringer's solution-soaked sterile sponges until needed later as an autograft during shell closure.

Immediately subjacent to the rectus muscle is the coelomic membrane and the twin thin-walled sinus-like ventral abdominal veins. Incise between these structures and enter the coelomic cavity, as in higher vertebrates. Most of the visceral organs are rather tightly bound by mesenteric, mesovarial, and other fibrous attachments; thus, they may be difficult to exteriorize and require working within the coelom. The urinary bladder and gravid oviducts are exceptions.

After correction of the problem and repair of any visceral incisions, close the coelomic membrane with absorbable sutures. If the coelomic membrane has been torn during the initial celiotomy and cannot be sutured, it can be left unclosed without untoward effect except for the possibility of postoperative adhesions. Once the flap has been replaced properly, the visceral organs are kept in place without risk of wound dehiscence and evisceration.

Exposure of the coelomic cavity to the environment does not necessarily impair respiration in chelonians. These animals do not have a functional diaphragm, and their respiratory gases are exchanged with the help of contractions of the intrapulmonary smooth muscle and extrapulmonary skeletal muscles, particularly those of the brachial girdle.

In instances of traumatic injury, the patient usually remains active and probably should be sedated with an anesthetic agent such as ketamine hydrochloride or alphoxolone-alphadolone acetate to facilitate the repair.

APPLICATION OF EPOXY RESIN-IMPREGNATED FIBERGLASS PATCHES

Fiberglass patches are applied to chelonians as follows:

1. Autoclaved fiberglass patches cut in a round or oval shape are selected in a size that will permit at least 1.5 to 3.0 cm to extend beyond the edge of the bony defect. Square patches tend to unravel or pucker along their edges and should be avoided.

2. The surface of the shell is cleansed with several applications of surgical scrub, sterile water or saline rinses, and then it is dried with sterile sponges, afterwhich ether or acetone is applied and allowed to air dry completely. This last application will help ensure that a firm bond will form between the outer shell and the epoxy resin-impregnated fiberglass patch.

3. Freshly prepared rapid polymerizing epoxy resin (5-Minute Epoxy Cement[R]-Devcon, or an equivalent product) is applied to the *periphery* of the shell defect and extended

approximately 2 cm. *Care must be taken not to invade the defect or touch its edges.* This is particularly important, for if the epoxy resin is permitted to become interposed between the edges of the incision, it will impede bone healing.

4. The first fabric patch is positioned over the hole so that its margins contact the freshly applied epoxy resin, and the resin is gently but thoroughly worked into the interstices of the patch while the patch is stretched taughtly over the hole.

5. When the first coat of epoxy resin has polymerized, the central portion of the fiberglass cloth patch can be given a light coating of epoxy resin. This coating should be only enough to moisten the fabric—not enough to drip through into the defect and coelomic cavity. Several thin coats are more desirable than a single thick one. One means for ascertaining the degree of penetration into the weave of the fabric is that when well permeated, the fiberglass cloth becomes nearly transparent and loses most of its woven appearance. If the woven texture of the fabric can still be seen after epoxy has been applied, it denotes an insufficient epoxy penetration and bonding; the entire patch should be removed and a new one substituted. These patches *must* be absolutely air- and watertight to prevent invasion by pathogenic microorganisms.

6. After this first layer has polymerized, additional epoxy-impregnated patches may be applied in the same manner until the desired thickness and strength have been achieved. In most cases, two layers of fiberglass fabric and epoxy resin are sufficient to repair surgical incisions and traumatic wounds effectively.

Although some exothermic heat of polymerization is produced as the epoxy resin cures, it is dissipated over the surface of the patches and will not harm the subjacent living tissues. When the components in the two-part epoxy kit are used in a ratio of 1:1, the time required for polymerization, as determined by generation of heat and the formation of a gel, is approximately 3 to 5 minutes. Within another 4 or 5 minutes, the surface of the patch will lose its tackiness and becomes hard. A light wiping of the cured surface with diethyl ether between coats of epoxy resin improves the bond between them.

After the last coat of epoxy has completely polymerized and lost its tackiness, a light spraying of the patched surface with aerosol vegetable oil pan coating (Pam[R], or its generic equivalent) will prevent the new patch from adhering to newspaper or other substrates before placing the chelonian back into ventral recumbency.

When a piece of devascularized bone is to be positioned and serves as an autograft, the technique is essentially identical to that described above. The autograft is bonded first to the *central* portion of the fabric patch with epoxy resin. The peripheral portion of the patch will be bonded in a later step. Once the first application of epoxy resin has polymerized, the process proceeds as for the application of a simple patch. Fresh resin must not drip into or between the autograft edges and the edges of the shell defect because the epoxy will serve as a barrier to osteogenic bridging.

Although a number of other resins are available, I prefer to use clear products because they are readily available, inexpensive, cosmetically acceptable, and highly resistant to abrasion and moisture. Dental acrylic plastics, hoof-repair compounds, and colored polyester resins also can be used, but they are opaque and do not possess the abrasion resistance of the fiberglass-epoxy resin laminates. Dental acrylic may be useful in situations where the repair must come into intimate contact with moist, soft tissues. This material is non-toxic and polymerizes without producing signficant heat of polymerization.

If a totally natural-appearing repair is essential, finely ground shell can be added to the final layer of epoxy resin. Moreover, the still slightly soft surface of the patch can be embossed or etched with an engraving tool. Alternatively, a piece of natural shell with deeply defined growth rings or striae can be used as a stamp with which to imprint a pattern of concentric rings.

Occasionally, interfragmentary wiring and plating of severely collapsed shell fractures must be done to repair massive trauma resulting from crushing injuries. If evidence of paralysis or posterior limb paresis, or both, is present, and a neurological examination reveals spinal cord injury, the prognosis is unfavorable. In such a case, euthanasia should be considered because it is a humane alternative to severe chronic debility. Dorsoventral and lateral radiographic views aid in defining the extent of spinal injuries.

Complete healing may require two or more years. The patches may be left in situ for the life of an adult tortoise or turtle. However, in a young, growing chelonian, these patches will interfere with growth, which occurs at the interfaces between adjacent bony plates or scutes; the patch may have to be removed from those areas immediately overlying the expanding growth rings. This may be accomplished as early as six months after the intitial repair. The cured resin-fiberglass is carefully routed away with a hand-held motorized rotary file or bur. **A word of caution:** the dust created by this motorized routing procedure can be **extremely** irritating to the ophthalmic, respiratory, and gastrointestinal epithelium in man (and, presumably, animals). It may, in fact, even be equally carcinogenic as asbestos and gypsum fibers. Therefore, suitable protective garb should be worn when the procedure is performed. A simple disposable respiratory mask and eye goggles or safety spectacles usually are adequate for this; if a vacuum hood is available, this would be an ideal situation for protecting the patient and its veterinary surgeon.

AMPUTATIONS

When the digits of crocodilians, lizards, and chelonians must be removed, they are best amputated immediately adjacent to the fleshy portion of the manus or pes; e.g., at the phalangeal-metacarpal/metatarsal joints. Similarly, the forelimb is removed via scapulo-humeral disarticulation; the hind limb is amputated at the coxofemoral joint. These methods will ensure that no stump remains to be abraded and becomes a chronic problem. The cosmetic results that are achieved by these techniques are quite satisfactory and usually are acceptable even in animals on public display. The operative techniques are very similar to those employed with higher vertebrates. Generally, postoperative dressings are unnecessary unless occlusive pressure is desired to control capillary blood loss and seroma formation. A small-bore Penrose drain can be inserted if necessary.

CRYOSURGERY

Cryosurgical techniques should be considered where conventional surgical excision is impracticable or inappropriate.

Examples of such indications are some neoplastic and non-neoplastic lesions arising from the skull or mandible. Such lesions may not be amenable to complete sharp surgical extirpation and may recur. Others may leave massive tissue defects which may not be coverable by available skin. Highly vascular lesions are best managed with cryosurgery. Some broad-based or highly invasive inflammatory lesions and some oral tumors are particularly appropriate for cryosurgical extirpation.

After obtaining specimens for histopathologic examination and/or microbiological culture, the lesion(s) are intermittently deeply frozen and thawed for at least two or three cycles. This freezing is accomplished by applying cryosurgical instruments which have been cooled with liquid nitrogen. Smaller dermal lesions can be super chilled by applying a stream of liquid nitrogen from a disposable aerosol container fitted with a long, thin spout or nozzle (PCG 12 nitrous oxide Cryo-Gun[R] or Freon 12 (DuPont) in the form of Freez-it[R]- (Chemtronics, Inc., Hauppauge, NY 11788). Alternatively, liquid nitrogen can be held for a few hours in a closed vacuum bottle and applied with a cotton-tipped applicator for three freeze-thaw cycles. The frozen tissue undergoes aseptic necrosis and sloughs, leaving a healing bed of neofibrous granulation tissue which usually heals well.

RADIOFREQUENCY ELECTROSURGERY

The use of fully filtered and fully or partially rectified current for precise surgery in reptiles has been demonstrated by several veterinary surgeons and has been shown to offer several advantages over conventional sharp dissection/excision techniques. The unit that has received the greatest acceptance is the Surgitron F.F.P.F.(R) (Ellman, 1135 Railroad Avenue, Hewlett, NY 11567 U.S.A.; 1-800-835-5355). The use of radiofrequency electrosurgery permits essentially bloodless technique, extreme precision, and enhanced primary healing. It is particularly valuable for operating upon friable and/or highly vascular tissues. The incisions created with these instruments are dry and the adjacent tissues are relatively unaffected by the passage of the radiofrequency current.

REPAIR OF MAXILLOFACIAL AND MANDIBULAR FRACTURES

Occasionally, chelonians, particularly terrestrial tortoises, suffer traumatic injuries to their jaws. The majority of these injuries are the result of automobile accidents. Because of the thinness of the bones involved and their propensity to comminute, these fractures are often severely compounded, severely displaced, and usually contaminated.

Simple drilling and wiring of the bone and keratin-covered tissue fragments fails to offer sufficient stabilization. Recently, I have had the opportunity to employ a combination of both internal and external fixation methods together to stabilize maxillofacial and mandibular fractures in these animals.

The surgical goal is to bring the multiple fracture fragments together, using sterile technique. After the fracture site has been thoroughly cleansed and prepared for aseptic surgery, the largest fragments are brought into apposition and wired together using small drill holes and stainless steel suture wire. The wires are passed through fine drill holes and thence into the bevelled end of a disposable hypodermic needle that is itself passed through a small hole in an opposite bone fragment. The needle is then withdrawn gently with the length of wire until both have passed through the far side. This technique makes the mating of the two ends of the wires relatively simple and straightforward. The wires are either tied or twisted on the *outside* of the jaw(s) in such a fashion that the wires lie flat against the outer surface. Once all of the fragments have been fixed into position and held firmly in place, the wires are encased in one or more layers of rapid polymerizing self-curing plasticized polymethymethacrylate resin commonly used in the dental profession for repairing dentures (Jet Denture Repair Acrylic, Product 1223; Lang Dental Mfg. Co., Inc., P.O. Box 969, 175 Messner Drive, Wheeling Illinois, 60090 USA; Fastray, Harry J. Bosworth Co., 7227 N. Hamlin Avenue, Skokie, Ilinois, 60076, U.S.A.).

To illustrate the technique, I have selected a case of severe, but typical multiple fractures involving the maxillary and mandibular bones of a California desert tortoise, *Xerobates agassizi*, whose rostrum and the anterior third of the mandible had been run over by an automobile. One orbit had collapsed and the eye appeared to have been destroyed. The contralateral eye was intact but severely bruised. Parenthetically, had both eyes been lost, I probably would not have performed the surgical repair because being a sight feeder, this animal would have had to depend on being hand fed for the balance of its life. However, with monocular vision it should be able to feed once the fractures have healed. The maxilla and rostral premaxilla had sustained at least six displaced fractures with various degrees of anatomical displacement.

A latex rubber dam or a piece of disposable latex surgeon's glove is placed onto the skin surface immediately beneath the fixation wires. This dam confines the acrylic plastic and permits its molding. The poly methylmethacrylate is built up until the desired thickness and shape is attained. Polymerization is almost instant, rarely requiring more than one minute.

In the case of compound fractures, the patient is placed upon an bacterio*cidal*, rather than a bacterio*static*, antibiotic. My colleagues and I now administer enrofloxacin (Baytril[R]-Mobay) as the antibiotic of choice at a dosage of 10 mg/kg/24 hours. This drug is available in both oral and injectable forms; Mader (1991, pers. communication) reported that the injectable form is effective when given orally as drops. Under most circumstances, the drug is given to the tortoises orally. This is done because the injectable form tends to produce significant muscle pain and even myonecrosis at the site of deep intramuscular injection. An alternative medication, clindamycin HCl (Antirobe[R]-Upjohn), is available in an oral suspension form which make its administration to animals with maxillo-facial injuries easier than tablets or capsules. If necessary, a pharyngostomy and feeding tube emplacement can be performed to more readily maintain a patient's fluid, caloric, and medication needs. Once the fractures have been adequately stabilized, this oral dosing is easily accomplished by the owners, after they have been shown how to open their pet's mouth and administer the tablets.

The process of healing usually is monitored radiographically during the 8-to-12-months following surgical repair. Once the maxillo-facial and/or mandibular fractures have healed sufficiently, the acrylic plastic and wires are removed by cutting the latter. If necessary, the wire and acrylic splintage can be left in situ indefinitely unless the patient is an actively growing juvenile—in which case healing usually is rapid.

When last seen for evaluation, it had been 23 months after the trauma and surgical repair. The mandibular and maxillary fractures were healed and the tortoise had been eating by itself for several months and the eye, which I thought had been destroyed, was functional; both direct and consensual reflexes were intact and the animal could locate food items.

OVERGROWN MOUTHPARTS AND CLAWS

Overgrown horny mouthparts of chelonians can be trimmed with a hand-held rotating saw blade held in the chuck of a Dremel MotoTool or similar instrument. Less severe deformities can be trimmed with sandpaper or an emory board, file, or equivalent abrasive device. Similarly, overgrown claws should be trimmed with an appropriate clipper or shears, depending upon the size of the claws.

SUTURELESS TREATMENT FOR SKIN LACERATIONS AND ABRASIONS

Often, snakes and lizards fail to adjust to the conditions of captivity and develop sterotypical behavior patterns characterized by "pacing" along the perimeters of their cages. Others may fail to recognize the limitation of the cage's transparent walls and, because of this, damage their rostral scales by crashing into the transparent material. Yet others, particularly water dragon lizards and some iguanas, damage their rostra when they dive from an overwater branch into a too shallow container of water.

Most of these traumatic injuries can be prevented by providing a visual barrier that the animal can see; water depth should be adequate to meet the needs of each animal.

These lesions can be treated by providing a "breathable" dressing that protects the traumatized site and permits the damaged tissue to heal. One product that has proven particularly practical is New Skin[R]-Medtech Laboratories, Inc. Jackson, WY 83001. This product contains a 6.7% alcoholic solution of pyroxylin, oil of cloves, and 8-hydroxyquinoline and is useful for providing temporary protection of ulcerative carapacial and plastral lesions also. New Skin is inexpensive and readily available as an over-the-counter item at most drugstores. One or several layers of this liquid dressing are applied to the site, allowing a few minutes for the material to dry between layers. New Skin can also be applied over skin sutures to protect them from moisture-induced maceration or to provide the line of incision additional support, and to minor rodent bites.

NONSURGICAL RETRIEVAL OF GASTRIC FOREIGN BODIES

Although not always a totally voluntary act, ingestion of a surprising variety of foreign bodies is seen in some captive reptiles, particularly chelonians (e.g., mata mata turtles), large lizards (e.g., monitors), and crocodilians. Many of these items do not cause clinical signs and are discovered only when radiographs are made for some unrelated reason.

If the animal's size permits insertion of a gastroscope or similar endoscopic device, the object often can be snared with a small loop of monofilament nylon or stainless steel utilizing a technique with one end fixed and with the other end attached to a long flexible probe or rod.

Alternative methods for retrieval include flexible probes equipped with small permanent magnets (for ferrous metallic objects) and four-pronged flexible "pick-up" devices used by mechanics and electronic technicians. This device is passed through the mouth and esophagus with its prongs closed. When the plunger is depressed, the prongs open to surround the object. When the plunger is released, the prongs close and grasp the foreign body, which can then be withdrawn through the endoscope without injuring delicate soft tissues. Care must be taken to avoid accidentally grasping the esophageal and/or gastric mucosa. A similar technique has proven useful for extracting some urocystoliths from lizards via the cloaca. At the time that this manuscript was being written, the cost for this device in a local hardware store was $1.95; this modest price makes it equivalent to many disposable medical products.

These methods can be used to remove ingested nails, screws, hairpins, pieces of glass or plastic, metal bottle caps, toys, etc.—the full array of odd objects that find their way into the captive environment of these animals is nearly limitless. Often, these ferrous metallic objects can be extracted from the stomach with a flexible shaft-mounted permanent magnet, similar to the pick-up tool noted above.

DYSTOCIA

Unlike mammals, when reptiles experience difficulty in delivering their eggs or young, it is not because of primary uterine inertia or hypocalcemia but, rather, it usually is due to malformed or abnormally large eggs. Therefore, while it might not induce any physiological disorders, the use of calcium generally is not necessary as an adjunct to the injection of oxytocin or other posterior pituitary hormone. When used to induce oviductal contractions, oxytocin is administered at a dosage rate of 1–2 international units/100g of body weight. Please note: while this dosage has been used widely for relatively small reptiles, much lower dosages are appropriate for larger animals. Recently, investigations into the comparative physiological effects of oxytocin and arginine vasotocin (AVT), lysine vasotocin (LVT), and aminosuberic arginine vasotocin (AsuAVT) in gravid reptiles have shown that vasotocin is substantially (>10 times) more effective, and requires less time to exhibit its smooth muscle effects on the oviduct. These three separate vasotocin products are available from Sigma Chemical Co. In the study cited (Lloyd, M. *Proc. IV Int. Coll. Pathol. Med. Reptiles & Amphib.*, Bad Nauheim, Germany, 27–29 September, 1991, Pp. 299–306), Lloyd recommended a treatment regimen of 0.2–0.5 ml/kg Calphosan given 30 to 120 minutes prior to the injection of arginine vasotocin at a dosage of 0.01 to 1.0 mcg/kg intravenously; if necessary, an intramuscular or intracoelomic injection can be employed, but the intravenous route is preferable. Confining the injected reptile in a moderately warm and secluded cage was recommended by Lloyd.

Warm water baths may also help induce gravid or pregnant reptiles to deliver their eggs or young. In those instances where conservative medical treatment fails to cause oviductal evacuation, the dystocia may have to be relieved by surgical removal of retained ova or embryos.

SPECIAL BANDAGING TECHNIQUES

Applying bandages to lizards and crocodilians usually can be accomplished using routine methods applicable to other quadripeds. However, employing occlusive dressings to snakes often can be an exercise in futility because of snakes' ability to crawl out of most conventional dressings. Where applicable, and especially when dealing with lesions caudal to the cloacal vent, I have found the use of *nonlubricated* condoms extremely useful because once the open end is taped to the snake patient's skin, the condom is usually very well tolerated. Typically, a moist dressing containing an antibiotic or antiseptic such as silver sulfadiazine cream or other product is applied to the affected epidermis, as well as to the interior of the reservoir end of the condom before it is drawn over the tail and attached to the skin with a length of Elasticon(R) or similar elastic tape. In my practice, these medication-filled condoms have become standard therapy for several conditions that heretofore had been extremely difficult to treat.

In order to prevent cotton cast padding or gauze sponge material from slipping or becoming dislodged from intimate contact with reptilian skin, apply a light coat of tincture of Benzoin or New Skin(R) (Medtech Laoratories, Inc., Jackson,

Wy 83001 USA), and place the padding or gauze while the Benzion or New Skin$^{(R)}$ are still tacky.

TREATMENT METHODS

Injection sites are important in reptiles because of the renal portal vascular drainage from the caudal half of the body. Whenever possible, intramuscular injections of aminoglycosides and other drugs which may be nephrotoxic should be made into the muscles in the cranial half of the body. When making intracoelomic injections, the hypodermic needle need only be inserted to a depth that will ensure its penetration through the coelomic membrane. Deeper penetration is not necessary and risks injury to delicate intracoelomic structures. Sites for intravenous injections can be employed for venous sampling also.

Treatments that require soaking can best be accomplished by sandwiching the patient between clean cloth towels saturated with the medication solution. A foam box is used to help conserve warmth when the entire container is placed upon a heating pad.

Retained tertiary spectacle shields can be most easily softened and loosened before physical removal by applying a drop or two of sterile contact lens wetting solution such as SoacLens$^{(R)}$ (Alcon), followed by moisturizing with warm water for 5–10 minutes. Similarly, the surfactant qualities of SoacLens can be put to good advantage in helping to loosen dried, adhered shreds of retained skin in cases of dysecdysis. If contact lens wetting solution is unavailable, a substitute can be made by adding 4.0 ml dioctyl sodium sulfosuccinate and 1–2 drops mild dishwashing detergent to 120 ml tap water. After applying any of these solutions to the retained epidermis, allow 2–3 minutes for complete penetration before physically lifting them free.

EGG INCUBATION METHODS

Generally, most reptile eggs can be incubated by placing them in a medium consisting of slightly moistened sphagnum moss, vermiculite, of a mixture of clean, salt-free sand and vermiculite. Eggs from semiaquatic turtles and lizards, such as water dragons, require a more moist incubation medium; desert-dwelling tortoises, lizards, and most snakes require less moist nesting material. Incubation temperatures and times vary widely among reptiles, but usually an incubation temperature of 27–32.5°C (80.6 to 90.5°F) is adequate to facilitate embryonic development. Incubation times can vary between only two or three weeks to several months, depending upon the species and temperatures.

Please Note: for the sake of brevity in this book, I have deleted the illustrations and most of the literature sources cited in my 1991 two-volume text, Biomedical and Surgical Aspects of Captive Reptile Husbandry. Interested readers may obtain references from that book. However, in instances where literature is cited from sources that were published since the release of my 1991 two-volume text, the appropriate authorship attribution and publication have been included.

TABLE 17
PARENTERAL AND ORAL ANTIBIOTICS USED IN REPTILES

GENERIC NAME PRODUCT NAME	SOURCE	ROUTE	FREQUENCY	DOSAGE	REMARKS/ PRECAUTIONS
Acyclovir Zovirax(R)	Wellcome	Topically	s.i.d. b.i.d.	— —	6
Amikacin sulfate (Amikin(R)) (Amiglyde-V(R))	Bristol Bristol	IM IM	s.i.d. 72 hrs 96 hrs	80 mg/kg 2.5 mg/kg 2.25 mg/kg	N, PF 2 5
Amoxicillin (Amoxi-drops(R))	Beecham	O	s.i.d. b.i.d.	22.0 mg/kg	
Ampicillin trihydrate (Polyflex(R))	Bristol	O SC IM	s.i.d. b.i.d.	3–6 mg/kg	
Benzathine penicillin (Flocillin(R))	Bristol	IM	varies w/temperature 48–96 hours	10,000 units total penicillin activity/kg	
(Bicillin(R)) fortified	Wyeth	IM	repeat 48–96 hours	same	

GENERIC NAME PRODUCT NAME	SOURCE	ROUTE	FREQUENCY	DOSAGE	REMARKS/ PRECAUTIONS
Carbenicillin disodium (Geopen[R])	Roerig	IM IV	s.i.d. b.i.d.	50–100 mg/kg initially; 50–75 mg/kg thereafter	PF
Cephaloridine (Loridine[R])	Elanco	IM SC	b.i.d.	10 mg/kg	N, PF
Cephalothin sodium (Keflin[R])	Bristol	IM	b.i.d.	40–80 mg/kg in divided doses	
Cefotaxime (Claforan[R])	Hoechst-Roussel	IM	s.i.d.	20–40 mg/kg	
Chloramphenicol (Chloromycetin[R])	Parke-Davis	IM IV	b.i.d.	10–15 mg/kg in divided doses	N
Clindamycin HCl (tablets and suspension) (Antirobe[R])	Upjohn	O	b.i.d.	2.5–5.0 mg/kg	
Dihydrostreptomycin sulfate	Several sources	IM	s.i.d. b.i.d.	5 mg/kg	N, PF

Drug	Manufacturer	Route	Interval	Dose	Notes
Doxycycline calcium syrup (Vibramycin(R))	Pfizer	O	s.i.d.	1 mg/kg	
Enrofloxacin (Baytril(R))	Mobay	O IM	s.i.d. s.i.d.	7.5–10.0 mg/kg 7.5–10.0 mg/kg (may be diluted with sterile NS to reduce tissue irritation)	—
Gentamicin sulfate (Gentocin(R))	Schering	IM SC IM	q 48 hrs q 72 hrs q 96 hrs	10.0 mg/kg 2.5 mg/kg 1.75 mg/kg	N, PF 1 2 5
Kanamycin sulfate (Kantrex(R))	Bristol	IV IM wound irrig.	s.i.d. b.i.d. in divided doses	10–15 mg/kg	N, PF
Ketoconazole (Nizoral(R))	Janssen	O	q 24–32 hrs	10–30 mg/kg	only 1 ref. available for tortoises @30 mg/kg
Lincomycin (Lincocin(R))	Upjohn	IM	s.i.d. b.i.d.	6 mg/kg	N, PF
Metronidazole@ Flagyl(R)	Searle	O	s.i.d.	12.5–40 mg/kg	

GENERIC NAME PRODUCT NAME	SOURCE	ROUTE	FREQUENCY	DOSAGE	REMARKS/ PRECAUTIONS
Oxytetracycline (Liquamycin(R)) injectable intramuscular	Pfizer	IV IM	s.i.d.	6–10 mg/kg	—
Piperacillin (Pipracil(R))	Lederle	IM	s.i.d.	50–100 mg/kg	PF
Potassium pencillin G	many	IM IV SC	b.i.d.- t.i.d.	10,000– 20,000# units/kg	
Streptomycin sulfate	many	IM	s.i.d.- b.i.d.	10 mg/kg	N, PF
Sulfadimethoxine (Bactrovet(R))	Pitman-Moore	IV IM O	s.i.d.	90 mg/kg 1st day; 45 mg/kg 2d–6th days	N, PF
Sulfamethazine concentrate	Merck	O	s.i.d. s.i.d.	60–90 mg/kg 1st day; 45 mg/kg 2nd–5th day	
Sulfaquinoxyline concentrate	Merck	O	s.i.d.	0.04% in drinking water	

Ticarcillin (Ticar[R])	Beecham	IM	s.i.d.	50–100 mg/kg	PF
Tobramycin	Eli Lily	IM	q 48 hrs	10 mg/kg	N, PF 3, 4
Trimethroprim sulfadiazine (Tribrissen[R]) 24% Susp. Inj. (DiTrim[R])	Coopers Animal Health Syntex	IM IM	s.i.d. s.i.d.	10–20 mg/kg 10–20 mg/kg	PF PF
Trimethroprim sulfamethoxazole	Wellcome	O	s.i.d.	10–30 mg/kg of combined drug*	PF

NOTE: because reduced ambient and, thus, body temperature in reptiles greatly influences the absorption and clearance of many drugs, it is imperative that these animals are kept sufficiently warm during the time that they are being treated with chemotherapeutic drugs. This is particularly germane with the aminoglycosides. Supplemental warmth also enhances the action of these drugs and it will also diminish the likelihood that toxic levels will accumulate. Moreover, the increased body temperature will help augment the synthesis of immunoglobulins. Similarly, it is extremely important to maintain hydration during antibiotic therapy.

LEGEND
1. Nonscaled chelonian dosage
2. Nonscaled snake and lizard dosage
3. Nonscaled aquatic & semiaquatic turtle dosage
4. Nonscaled terrestrial chelonian dosage

5. Nonscaled crocodilian dosage
6. Human dose; reptilian dose has not been established

s.i.d. = once daily
b.i.d. = twice daily
t.i.d. = three times daily
q.i.d. = four times daily

* potassium ion excess may cause cardiac arrest at a high dosage or if injected too rapidly intravenously.

* = dosage based on trimethroprim fraction

@ this dosage used when metronidazole is administered as an adjunct drug together with other antibiotics, especially when treating an anaerobic infection, or when given as an immunostimulant. The dosage is higher when treating protozoan infections.

IM = administered by intramuscular injection
IV = administered by intravenous injection
SC = administered by subcutaneous injection
O = administered orally

PF = parenteral fluid supplementation recommended
N = potentially nephrotoxic; should be injected in the cranial half of the body; maintain adequate renal perfusion by supplementing fluids
I = may induce pain & inflammation may occur at injection sites

TABLE 18
MISCELLANEOUS DRUGS USED IN CAPTIVE REPTILES

GENERIC NAME	SOURCE	ROUTE	FREQUENCY	DOSAGE	REMARKS
Aminophylline	Searle	IM; supository	As needed	2–4 mg/kg as req'd	
Amphotericin-B	Squibb	slow IV; O; Nebulized with oxygen	2–3 time weekly	0.5 mg/kg	highly nephrotoxic; can be used in combination w/ketoconazol
Ascorbic acid	many	IM, IV	Varies	None established	
Arginine Vasotocin	Sigma	IV, Intra-coelomic	Varies	0.01–1.0 micrograms/kg	far greater dosages have been reported
Aminosuberic Arginine Vasotocin	Sigma	same	Varies	same	
Lysine Vasotocin	Sigma	same	Varies	same	
Atropine sulfate	many	IM, IV, SC, O	As needed	0.04 mg/kg	see glyco-pyrrolate

GENERIC NAME	SOURCE	ROUTE	FREQUENCY	DOSAGE	REMARKS
Calcitonin Calcimar(R)	Roerer	SC	t.i.d.	1.5 Int. U/kg	also give fluids IV or IC @ 10–15 ml/kg daily to enhance diuresis
Calcium gluconate injectable U.S.P.	Parke-Davis	IV, IM	As needed	500 mg/kg in divided doses; admin. slowly if IV	
Calcium glucobionate	Sandoz	O	s.i.d./b.i.d.	3.5 gm/kg	
Calcium gluconate 23%	TechAmerica	O	2–3 times weekly	0.5–1.0 ml/kg; use with oral vitamin D-3	
Calcium lactate + Calcium glycerophosphate	Carlton; Burns-Biotec	IM, O	as needed	0.2–0.5 ml/kg (5 mg/ml)	
Cimetidine Tagamet(R)	Smith-Kline Beckman	IM, O	b.i.d./q.i.d.	4 mg/kg*	

Cyanocobalamin	many	IM, SC	Not established	Not established
Hydroxycobalamin	many	IM, SC	Not established	10–2,000 mcg, depending upon body weight
Dexamethasone (Azium[R])	Schering & generic	IM, IV	As needed	0.625–0.125 mg/kg
Entromycin	Pitman-Moore	O	s.i.d.	1.25 ml/liter of drinking water or as a dredge
Flunixin meglumine (Banamine[R])	Schering	IV	s.i.d./b.i.d.	0.1–0.5 mg/kg 1–2 days
Furosemide (Lasix[R])	National	IV, IM	As needed	5 mg/kg PF
Furoxone[R] suspension	Eaton	O	s.i.d.	25–40 mg/kg
Glycopyrrolate (Robinul-V[R])	Robins	IV, IM	preanesthetic	10 micrograms/kg (0.050 ml/kg) Preferable to atropine sulfate
Ketoconazole Nizoral[R]	Jannsen	O	s.i.d. 24–32 hrs	10–30 mg/kg tortoises: 30 mg/kg

GENERIC NAME	SOURCE	ROUTE	FREQUENCY	DOSAGE	REMARKS
Methischol(R)	U.S. Vitamin & Pharm.	O	As needed	Not established	
Metronidizole Flagyl(R)	Searle	O	single dose	12.5–50 mg/kg	For appetite stimulation, not as a parasiticide, antibiotic, or immuno-stimulant; see dosage for antibiotic and parasiticidal dosages.
Oxytocin U.S.P. (see Aminosuberic arginine, and Lysine vasotocin also)	Many	IM	As needed	1–2 units / 100 g scaled for larger animals	
Prednisolone sodium succinate (Solu-Delta Cortef(R))	Upjohn	IV, IM	As needed	5–10 mg/kg	

Ranitidine HCl (Zantac[R])	Glaxo	O	b.i.d.	12 mg/kg*
Sodium Iodide injectable	Burns-Biotec	IV O	Not established	0.25–3.0 ml
Stanzolol (Winstrol[R])	Winthrop	IM	Not established	Not established
Sucralfate (Carafate[R])	Marion	O	t.i.d./q.i.d.	500–1,000 mg/kg
Vitamin A (Aquasol-A[R])	U.S. Vitamin & Pharmaceutical	IM#, O	Not established	Not established 1.0–10,000 units, depending upon body weight & condition being treated; oral route preferred. 500 IU/kg suggested by Barten (1991)
Vitamin B Complex	Many	IM, SC, O	not established	0.25–0.50 mg/kg; 0.1 ml/kg
Vitamin D$_3$	Several	O	1–2 times weekly	varies widely; ex. 1–4 i.u./kg

GENERIC NAME	SOURCE	ROUTE	FREQUENCY	DOSAGE	REMARKS
Vitamin K	Many	IM	Not established	0.25–0.75 mg/kg	

Legend
PF = parenteral fluid supplementation recommended
* = canine dosage; should scale dose to body weight of reptile
❋ = intramuscular injection may induce necrotic dermatitis and skin sloughing, particularly in chelonians; oral dosing advised

TABLE 19
TOPICAL OINTMENTS, SPRAYS, AND SOLUTIONS USED ON REPTILES

PRODUCT	SOURCE
Alupent 5% solution	Boehringer Ingelheim
Betadine Ointment	Purdue-Frederick
Betadine Scrub	Purdue-Frederick
Betadine Solution	Purdue-Frederick
Cromalyn Aerosol	Fisons
Dermafur Ointment	Eaton
Dermalog Ointment	Maurry
Furacin Ointment	Eaton
Furacin Solution	Eaton
Gentocin Durafilm Ophthalmic Solution	Schering
Gentocin Ophthalmic Solution	Schering
Kymar Ointment	Roche via Burns-Biotec
Metaprel 5% solution	Dorsey
Nasalcrom Nasal Solution	Fisons
New Skin Plastic Bandage	Medtech Laboratories
Nolvasan Scrub	Aveco
Nolvasan Solution	Aveco
Panalog Cream	Solvay
Panalog Ointment	Solvay
Povidone Iodine Solution	many generic products
Proventic Aerosol	Schering
Rezifilm Spray Bandage	Squibb
Silvadene Cream	Marion
Soac-Lens	Alcon
Sulfamylon Cream 8.5%	Wintrhop
Sulfa Urea Cream	Norden
Tinactin Ointment	Schering-Plough
Toptic Ointment	Corvel
Ventolin	Glaxo

TABLE 20
WOUND-IRRIGATING SOLUTIONS

PRODUCT	SOURCE
CHLORHEXIDINE DIACETATE* Nolvasan 0.5–1.0% solution	Aveco
POVIDONE IODINE SOLUTION Betadine Solution Generic 0.5–1.0% solution	Purdue-Frederick many
HYDROGEN PEROXIDE Hydrogen Peroxide, USP, 3% by volume 0.5–1.5% by volume	many
DAKIN'S SOLUTION Sodium Hypochlorite Solution household bleach 5.25% as a stock solution dilute to 0.5% final solution	many
ACETIC ACID (VINEGAR) dilute to 0.5% solution	many

* = preferred agent

TABLE 21
PARASITICIDES

PROTOZOA	GENERIC NAME	DOSAGE (mg/kg)	ROUTE	REFERENCE	COMMENTS
AMOEBAE & TRICHOMONADS	METRONIDAZOLE (Flagyl®-Searle)	125–250	O	Donaldson, et al. 1975	repeat in 10–14 days
		125–250	O	Frye, 1981	boid snakes; repeat in 2 wks
		12.5–40.0	O	Jacobson, 1991	some colubrid snakes
		275	O	Marcus, 1981	
		40–100	O	Funk, 1988	repeat in 2 weeks
	FLAGANASE 400	200		Cover & Hudson, 1988	repeat in 2 weeks
	(note lower dosage for appetite stimulation mentioned earlier)				
	Paromomycin	35–55;	O	Marcus, 1981	
	Park-Davis	25–100	O	Schweinfurth, 1970	
COCCIDIA	Sulfadiazine Many Mfrs.	75 1st day; 45 next 5 days	O	Funk, 1988	treat for 6 days
	Sulfamerazine Many Mfrs.	same	O	Funk, 1988	same

PROTOZOA	GENERIC NAME	DOSAGE (mg/kg)	ROUTE	REFERENCE	COMMENTS
	Sulfamethazine Many Mfrs.	75 in div. doses 1st day; 40 2nd–6th days 90 1st day; 45 next 5 days	O O	Frye, 1988 Funk, 1988	maintain hydration
	Sulfadimethoxine; Bactrovet^R; Albon^R	90 1st day; 45 next 5 days	O, IM IV	Frye, 1981	maintain hydration
	Sulfaquinoxyline Merck	75 in div. doses 1st day; 40 2nd–6th days	O, IM IV	Frye, 1981	maintain hydration
CRYPTOSPORIDIUM					
	Trimethroprim-Sulfadiazine Tribrissen$^{(R)}$ Coopers Animal Health DiTrim$^{(H)}$ Syntex	30–60 mg	O	Norton & Jacobson, 1989	may be toxic at this dosage

METAZOAN PARASITES PLATYHELMINTHS	GENERIC NAME	DOSAGE (mg/kg)	ROUTE	REFERENCE	COMMENTS
CESTODES	Bunamidine HCL (Scolaban[R]-Mobay)	25–50	O	Frye, 1981	Not more than every 2–3 weeks; do not use in cases of cardiac disease; repeat in 2 weeks
		50	O	Funk, 1988	
	Niclosamide (Yomesan[R]-Mobay)	150	O	Frye, 1981	
		150	O	Funk, 1988	
		300	O	Deakins, 1973	Repeat in 2 weeks
		165–200	O	Bush, 1974	
	Praziquantel (Droncit[R]-Mobay)	5–8 mg/kg	IM or O	Funk, 1988	Repeat in 2 weeks
	Febantel/ Praziquantel (Vercom Broad Spectrum[R] Anthelmintic Paste-Mobay)	580 (0.58 gm)	O	Miller, 1987	daily for 3 consecutive days
TREMATODES	Praziquantel Droncit[R]-Mobay)	8	O	Funk, 1988	repeat in 2 weeks

METAZOAN PARASITES	GENERIC NAME	DOSAGE (mg/kg)	ROUTE	REFERENCE	COMMENTS
PLATYHELMINTHS	Emetine HCL Injectable Eli Lilly	0.5	IM or SC	Frye, 1981	daily for 10 days
	Dithiazine iodide (Dizan[R]-Diamond)	20	O	Frye, 1981	will stain objects
	Dichlorvos (Task[R]-Shell)	12.5	O	Frye, 1981	
	Pyrantel pamoate Strongid-T[R]; Nemex-2[R]-Pfizer	5.0 (0.1 ml/kg)	O	Morgan, 1988	Repeat in 2 weeks
NEMATODES	Levamisol HCl (Tramisol[R]-Amer. Cyanamid)	5.0	IC	Frye, 1981	Intracoelomic inj. may be repeated in 2–3 weeks
	Levamisol Phosphate (Ripercol[R]-Amer. Cyanamid)	8.0	IC or SC	Frye, 1981	
		10.0	IC	Funk, 1988	Repeat in 2 weeks

Thiabendazole Thibenzole(R)-(Merck)	50.0	O	Frye, 1981	mix to liquid consistency.
	50.0	O	Marcus, 1981	
	50–100	O	Funk, 1988	Repeat in 2 weeks
Febantel/ Praziquantel (Vercom Broad Spectrum(R) Antehelmintic Paste-Mobay)	580 (0.58 gm)	O	Miller, 1987	daily for 3 consecutive days
Mebendazole (Merck)	20–25	O	Funk, 1988	Repeat in 2 weeks
Fenbendazole (Panacur(R)-Merck)	50–100	O	Funk, 1988	Repeat in 2 weeks
Ivermectin(R) Merck	200 mcg	IM	Funk, 1988	Repeat in 2 weeks (*) *DO NOT USE IN CHELONIANS*
	0.02 ml	O	several	

METAZOAN PARASITES	GENERIC NAME	DOSAGE (mg/kg)	ROUTE	REFERENCE	COMMENTS
PLATYHELMINTHS					
ECTOPARASITES	Ivermectin(R) Merck	200 mcg	IM	Funk, 1988	Repeat in 2 weeks (*) *DO NOT USE IN CHELONIANS*
		0.02 ml can also be employed as an enclosure spray	O	several	
	Vapona(R) No-Pest Strip- (Shell Chemical)	6.0 mm/10 cubic feet of cage space		Frye, 1981	Hang above cage or place in a vial with a perforated lid so animals can not come into contact with insecticide
	Almost any flea spray safe for kittens and puppies	apply sparingly to skin with a cloth slightly moistened with insecticidal spray			Do not use more than once weekly

Legend: O = *per os*; orally; IM = intramuscularly SC = subcutaneously IC = intracoelomically
mg = milligrams mcg = micrograms kg = kilograms (2.2 lbs); see conversion table on next page

s.i.d. = once daily
b.i.d. = twice daily
t.i.d. = three times daily
q.i.d. = four times daily

*Contraindicated in animals who have been given diazepam or who will be given diazepam within 10 days after being dosed with ivermectin.

TABLE 22
METRIC/ENGLISH/APOTHECARY CONVERSION VALUES

LINEAR MEASUREMENTS
1 millimeter = 0.039 inch
1 meter = 3.281 feet

1 inch = 25.4 millimeters
1 foot = 0.305 meter

VOLUMETRIC MEASUREMENTS
1 liter = 33.815 fluid ounces
1 liter = 1.057 quarts
1 liter = 0.264 gallon
1 liter = 1,000 milliliters
1 liter = 10 deciliters
1 deciliter = 100 milliliters

1 fluid ounce = 29.573 milliliters
1 fluid ounce = 0.3 liter
1 pint = 0.473 liter
1 quart = 0.946 liter
1 U.S. gallon = 3.785 liters
1 U.S. gallon = 128 ounces
   = 0.83 British Imperial gal.

1 British
Imperial gallon = 4.546 liters
   = 1.2 U.S. gal.

1 milliliter = 15–20 drops
5 milliliters = 1 teaspoon
3 teaspoons = 1 tablespoon
2 tablespoons = 1 ounce
1 teacup = 180 milliliters
1 glass = 240 milliliters
1 meas. cup = 240 milliliters (1/2 pint)

30 milliliters = 1 fluid ounce
473.2 milliliters = 1 pint
946 milliliters = 1 quart

MEASUREMENTS OF MASS

METRIC

1 microgram	=	0.001 milligram
1 milligram	=	0.035 ounce avoidup.
1 gram	=	1/454 pound
1 gram	=	1,000 milligrams
1 kilogram	=	2.205 pounds
1 kilogram	=	1,000 grams
1 mg/kg	=	0.454 mg/lb

AVOIDUPOIS

1 ounce (Av)	=	31.1 gram
1 pound	=	0.454 kilogram
	=	454 grams
1 mg/lb	=	2.2 mg/kg

APOTHECARY

1 grain = 60 mg (0.06 gm)
15 grainsz 1 gram

TABLE 23
kg/M^2/lb CONVERSIONS

kg	M^2	lbs	kg	M^2	lb
0.5	0.06	1.1	26	0.88	57.3
1	0.10	2.2	27	0.90	59.5
2	0.15	4.4	28	0.92	61.7
3	0.20	6.6	29	0.94	63.9
4	0.25	8.8	30	0.96	66.1
5	0.29	11.0	31	0.99	68.3
6	0.33	13.2	32	1.01	70.5
7	0.36	15.4	33	1.03	72.8
8	0.40	17.6	34	1.05	74.9
9	0.43	19.8	35	1.07	77.2
10	0.46	22.0	36	1.09	79.4
11	0.49	24.3	37	1.11	81.6
12	0.52	26.5	38	1.13	83.8
13	0.55	28.7	39	1.15	86.0
14	0.58	30.9	40	1.17	88.2
15	0.60	33.1	41	1.19	90.4
16	0.63	35.3	42	1.21	92.6
17	0.66	37.5	43	1.23	94.8
18	0.69	39.7	44	1.25	97.0
19	0.71	41.9	45	1.26	99.2
20	0.74	44.1	46	1.28	101.0
21	0.76	46.3	47	1.30	104.0
22	0.78	48.5	48	1.32	106.0
23	0.81	50.7	49	1.34	108.0
24	0.83	52.9	50	1.36	110.0
25	0.85	55.1			

TABLE 24
TEMPERATURE CONVERSION

Celsius Deg.	Fahr. Deg.	Celsius Deg.	Fahr. Deg.	Celsius Deg.	Fahr. Deg.
0	32.0	17	62.6	34	93.2
+1	33.8	18	64.4	35	95.0
2	35.6	19	66.2	36	96.8
3	37.4	20	68.0	37	98.6
4	39.2	21	69.8	38	100.4
5	41.0	22	71.6	39	102.2
6	42.8	23	73.4	40	104.0
7	44.6	24	75.2	41	105.8
8	46.4	25	77.0	42	107.6
9	48.2	26	78.8	43	109.4
10	50.0	27	80.6	44	111.2
11	51.8	28	82.4	45	113.0
12	53.6	29	84.2	46	114.8
13	55.4	30	86.0	47	116.6
14	57.2	31	87.8	48	118.4
15	59.0	32	89.6	49	120.2
16	60.8	33	91.4	50	122.0

for temperatures not listed above use the following formulae:

°Celsius to °Fahrenheit: $(°C)\left(\dfrac{9}{5}\right) + 32$

°Fahrenheit to °Celsius $1.8 \times °C + 32$
or $(°F - 32°)\left(\dfrac{5}{9}\right)$

APPENDIX A

REPTILE INFORMATION FORMS

CLIENT'S REPTILE HISTORY FORM #1

This form has been developed by us to serve you in a more efficient and practical way. These questions will aid our staff in the physical examination and evaluation of your reptile and allow Dr. Frye to make any recommendations necessary for the health and welfare of your reptile.

DATE _____
OWNER'S NAME _____
REPTILE'S NAME _____
TYPE OF REPTILE _____ SEX (if known) _____
AGE _____
WHO REFERRED YOU TO US _____
HOW LONG HAVE YOU OWNED THIS ANIMAL? _____
WHERE DID YOU OBTAIN IT? _____
IF KNOWN, IS IT CAPTIVE BRED OR WILD CAUGHT? _____
DO YOU OWN OTHER REPTILES? _____
WHAT SPECIES? _____
WHAT IS THIS REPTILE'S USUAL DIET? _____
DO YOU USE VITAMINS AND/OR MINERAL SUPPLEMENTS? IF SO PLEASE TELL US WHAT PRODUCTS OR ITEMS ARE USED _____
_____

WHAT, IN YOUR OPINION, IS THIS REPTILE'S MAJOR PROBLEM?
_____
_____
WHAT DO YOU BELIEVE MAY HAVE CAUSED THIS CONDITION?
_____
HOW LONG HAS YOUR REPTILE HAD THIS CONDITION?
_____
HAS THIS REPTILE BEEN EXPOSED TO OTHER REPTILES RECENTLY? _____
IS THERE ANY HISTORY OF PREVIOUS ILLNESS OR INJURY? __
_____
ARE THERE ANY MEDICATIONS YOUR REPTILE IS BEING GIVEN CURRENTLY? _____
IF SO, PLEASE IDENTIFY THE DRUG AND ITS DOSAGE _____
_____
WHAT IS YOUR REPTILE'S APPETITE CURRENTLY? _____
DO ITS STOOLS APPEAR NORMAL? _____
HAVE THERE BEEN ANY RECENT ADDITIONS TO YOUR COLLECTION? _____
IS THIS REPTILE NORMALLY KEPT BY ITSELF IN A CAGE OR ENCLOSURE? _____

Thank you for taking the time and effort to fill out this questionnaire. It will greatly facilitate our professional staff to evaluate the condition and husbandry of your reptile. Please feel free to ask any questions that may come to mind when your reptile is being examined. Remember, the questions you ask may be important; consequently we encourage any questions. COMMENTS: _____
_____

APPENDIX A

REPTILE HISTORY FORM #2

I. EPIDEMIOLOGIC DATA
   A. History of previous diseases in the area or collection.
   _____
   _____
   _____

   B. Morbidity and mortality among those animals at risk and/or affected with the condition under investigation.
   _____
   _____
   _____

   C. Rapidity of spread among the population at risk. ___
   _____
   _____

   D. Source of the animals within the entire population.
      1. Source and dates of all recent arrivals; length of quarantine period; history of losses due to diseases during quarantine. _____
      _____
      _____

      2. Previous history of diseases in animals obtained from same supplier. _____
      _____
      _____

   E. Food supplies, their sources, means of handling and storing prior to feeding, methods for presenting food items to the animals. _____
   _____
   _____

F. Water management and water delivery systems. _____
_____
_____

G. Waste management practices. _____
_____

H. Cage hygiene practices. _____
_____

   1. How often are cages cleaned? _____
_____

   2. What products are employed as disinfectants and at what dilutions? _____
_____

   3. Which personnel are involved? _____
_____

I. Pesticide application data. _____
_____

   1. What products were used? _____
_____

   2. Their dilution and expected residues. _____
_____

   3. Dates of application. _____
_____

   4. Personnel involved in their application. _____
_____

J. Census of other species present that could serve as reservoir hosts or vectors. _____
_____

K. Records of any temperature extremes prior to outbreak. _____

APPENDIX A

L. Miscellaneous.
   1. History of handling or display prior to the outbreak.

II. MACROSCOPIC AND MICROSCOPIC LESIONS AND CLINICAL SIGNS IN AFFECTED ANIMALS
   A. Special staining and/or histochemical techniques applied to tissue sections and/or exfoliative cytology/impression smears. _____

   B. Biochemical and clinical pathology tests of body fluids from affected individuals. _____

III. ISOLATION OF BACTERIAL, FUNGAL, AND/OR VIRAL AGENTS FROM TISSUES AND BODY FLUIDS
   A. May require special techniques employing varied culture media, incubation temperatures, and the manipulation of the incubation atmospheric oxygen concentration. _____

   B. Results of antibiotic sensitivity testing _____

IV. REPRODUCTION OF DISEASE IN HEALTHY REPTILES WITH ISOLATED AGENTS (fulfilling Koch's Postulates).
   A. This last criterion is optimum if one wishes to fulfill Koch's postulates in confirming that a particular pathogenic agent is responsible for inducing a particular disease. Because of the expense involved and/or the rarity of the animals, this last requirement often is justifiably omitted. If appropriate reptilian tissue culture material is available, cells may be inoculated with the suspected (viral) agent and subsequently examined for cytopathic effects and electronmicroscopic characterization.

   _____
   _____
   _____

V. CAGING, GENERAL HUSBANDRY INFORMATION FEEDING DATA (Diet, frequency of feeding, source of food, anything unusual, etc.) _____
_____

MEDICATION HISTORY (Drugs used, frequency, dates, route, length of course, etc.; pesticide usage. include product(s), frequency of application, personnel involved, etc.) _____
_____
_____
_____
_____

NARRATIVE DESCRIPTION OF OWNER/KEEPER (If available, attach written notes) _____

APPENDIX A

OTHER NOTES:

REPTILE PATHOLOGY ACCESSION FORM

SPECIES _____ ACCESSION NUMBER _____
BILLLING INFORMATION _____
BREED/TAXONOMY _____
DATE RECEIVED _____ DATE REPORTED _____
TAG, NAME OR IDENTIFICATION NUMBERS _____
SEX _____ AGE _____
CLINICIAN _____
ADDRESS _____
TELEPHONE/FAX NUMBERS _____ FAX _____
OWNER _____
ADDRESS _____
SPECIMEN(S): _____
DIED ____ HOURS ____ EUTHANATIZED BY _____
PRESERVATIVE _____
POSTMORTEM STATE _____
NUTRITIONAL STATE _____
LABORATORY WHERE HISTOLOGY PERFORMED: (VMTH; YOLO DIAG. X; PL;
ELECTROCARDIOGRAPHIC FINDINGS (please enclose tracings or photocopies):

_____
RADIOGRAPHS: _____
STAINED BLOOD FILM(S) OR OTHER BODY FLUIDS: _____

_____
NUMBER OF ANIMALS IN GROUP AFFECTED _____
DECALCIFICATION REQUIRED? _____
WEIGHT: (preferably in metric units) _____
GROSS NECROPSY OR PHYSICAL FINDINGS ("NSL" = no significant lesions; "NE" = not examined)

APPENDIX A

INTEGUMENT _____
PERITONEUM/COELOM _____
DIGESTIVE CANAL _____
LIVER AND GALLBLADDER _____
PANCREAS _____
SPLEEN _____
THYMUS _____
URINARY SYSTEM _____
GENITAL SYSTEM _____
PLEURA _____
RESPIRATORY SYSTEM _____
CARDIOVASCULAR SYSTEM _____
LYMPHATIC SYSTEM _____
MUSCULOSKELETAL SYSTEM _____
NERVOUS SYSTEM _____
OTHER ENDOCRINE ORGANS _____
BONE MARROW (site, color, consistency) _____
SPECIAL SENSE ORGANS _____
TENTATIVE DIAGNOSES (if any) _____
ACCESSION NUMBER _____
CAPTIVE HUSBANDRY INFORMATION (Where & when obtained, caging information, previous health problems with this animal or any others in same cage or group, if any) _____

_____
_____

FEEDING DATA (Diet, frequency of feeding, source of food, anything unusual, etc.) _____

_____
_____
_____

MEDICATION HISTORY (Drugs used, frequency, dates, route, length of course, etc.; pesticide usage. include product(s), frequency of application, personnel involved, etc.) _____
_____
_____
_____
_____

NARRATIVE DESCRIPTION OF OWNER/KEEPER (If available, attach written notes) _____
_____
_____
_____
_____
_____
_____

PHOTOMICROGRAPHS/PHOTOMACROGRAPHS MADE? (YES/NO) _____

PLEASE NOTE: If you wish to have the pathologist send you a copy of this pathology report by facsimile, please request this service by checking the box below and supplying your facsimile telephone number. A hard copy will also be sent via first class mail.

I/We request report sent via fax ☐ My fax number is _____

APPENDIX B

NONTOXIC AND TOXIC PLANTS

Many plants are nontoxic to reptiles and can be used safely for landscaping pet enclosures to make them more attractive and comfortable. Here is a list of suitable plants.

Some mildly irritating to profoundly toxic wild and cultivated plants are occasionally ingested by captive reptiles, particularly terrestrial tortoises. A partial list of the more common species that have been implicated in plant intoxications follows the nontoxic list.

NONTOXIC PLANTS SUITABLE FOR LANDSCAPING REPTILE ENCLOSURES

PLANT NAME

ABELIA (*Abelia grandiflora*)
AFRICAN VIOLET (*Saintpaulia ionantha*)
SWEET ALYSSUM (*Allyssum* sp.)
ASPERAGUS FERN (*Asperagus setaceus plumosus*)
ASTER (*Aster* sp.)
BABY TEARS (*Helxine soleirolii*)
BIRD'S NEST FERN (*Asplenium nidus*)
BOSTON FERN (*Nephrolepsis exalta*)
BOTTLE BRUSH (*Callistemom* sp.)
BOUGANVILLEA (*Bouganvillea* sp.)
BRIDAL VEIL (*Tripogandra multiflora*)

BROMELIADS (*Aechmea; Bilbergia; Cryptanthus; Vriesia*, etc.)
CACTUS, SPINELESS (*Astrophytum*)
CAMELLIA (*Camellia japonica*)
COLEUS (*Coleus* sp.)
CORN PLANT (*Dracaena fragrans*)
CREEPING CHARLIE (*Pilea nummulariifolia*)*
CROTON (*Codiaeum* SP.)
DRACAENA (*Dracaena* SP.)
EMERALD RIPPLE (*Peperomia caperata*)
EUGENIA (*Eugenia* sp.)
FUSCHIA (*Fuschia*)
GERANIUM (*Pelargonium* sp.)
HEN AND CHICKS SUCCULENT (*Echeveria imbricata*)
HIBISCUS (*Hibiscus rosa-sinensis*)
HOYA (*Hoya exotica*)
ICEPLANT (*Mesembryanthemum crystallinum*)
IMPATIENS (*Impatiens*)
JADE PLANT (*Crassula argentea*)
JAPANESE ARALIA (*Fatsia japonica*)
JASMINE (*Jasminum officinale; J. grandiflorum*)
LAVENDER (*Lavandula officinalis*)
MARIGOLD (*Calendula officinalis*)
MONKEY PLANT (*Ruellia makoyana*)
MOTHER OF PEARL (*Graptopetalum paraguayense*)
NATAL PLUM (*Carissa grandiflora*)
PAINTED NETTLE (*Coleus*)
PALMS (*Areca* sp.)
PAMPAS GRASS (*Cortaderia selloana*)
PARLOR PALM (*Chamaedorea elegans*)
PEPEROMIA (*Peperomia caperata*)
PETUNIA (*Petunia*)
PHOENIX (*Phoenix roebelenii*)
PIGGYBACK PLANT (*Tolmiea menziesii*)
PILEA (*Pilea* sp.)
PINK POLKA-DOT PLANT (*Hypoestes sanguinolenta*)
PONYTAIL PLANT (*Beaucarnea recurvata*)
PRAYER PLANT (*Maranta leuconeura*)

APPENDIX B

PURPLE PASSION; PURPLE VELVET (*Gynura aurantiaca*)
SPIDER PLANT (*Chlorophytum comosum*)
STAGHORN FERN (*Platycerium bifurcatum*)
SWEDISH IVY (*Plectranthus australis*)
TREE MALLOW (*Lavatera assurgentiflora*)
UMBRELLA PLANT (*Eriogonum umbrellum*)#
VELVET PLANT (*Gynura aurantiaca*)
WANDERING JEW (*Tradescantia albiflora*); and (*Zebrina pendula*)
WARNECKII (*Dracaena deremensis*)
WAX PLANT (*Hoya exotica*)
ZEBRA PLANT (*Calathea zebrina*)
ZINNIAS (*Zinnia* sp.)

---

*not to be confused with another "creeping Charlie," *Glecoma heteracea* which is toxic.
#not be confused with another "umbrella" plant, *Schefflera actinophylla* which is toxic.
Modified from a list of plants published by *Tortuga Gazette, 28* (1):9–10.

TOXIC PLANTS

PLANT NAME	TOXIC PORTION(S)
ACOKANTHERA	FLOWERS AND FRUIT
ACONITE (MONKSHOOD) (*Aconitum*)	ROOTS, FLOWERS, LEAVES, AND SEEDS
AFRICAN LILY (*Agapanthus*) sp.	FOLIAGE, BULB
ALGAE, BLUE-GREEN (*Mycrocystis*)	ALL PARTS
ALOE	SUCCULENT FOLIAGE
AMARYLLIS	BULB, STEM, FLOWER PARTS
AMSINCKIA (TARWEED)	FOLIAGE AND SEEDS
ANEMONE	LEAVES, FLOWERS
APPLE (*Malus*)	SEEDS (ONLY IF CRUSHED)
APRICOT (SEEDS ONLY) (*Prunus*)	INNER SEEDS
ARROWHEAD VINE (*Syngonium*)	FOLIAGE, FRUIT
AUTUMN CROCUS (*Colchicum*)	BULBS
AVOCADO (*Persea*)	FOLIAGE, FRUIT IN SOME CIRCUMSTANCES
AZALEA (*Rhododendron*)	FOLIAGE, FLOWERS
BANEBERRY (*Actaea*)	FOLIAGE, FRUITS
BEGONIA	TUBERS, FOLIAGE, BLOSSOMS
BELLADONNA (*Digitalis*)	BERRIES AND OTHERS PARTS
BETAL NUT PALM (*Areca catachu*)	ALL PARTS
BIRD OF PARADISE (*Strelitzia*)	FOLIAGE, FLOWERS, SEED PODS
BITTERSWEET NIGHTSHADE (*Solanum*)	BERRIES
BLACK LOCUST (*Robinia*)	BARK, SPROUTS, AND FOLIAGE
BLEEDING HEART (*Dicentra*)	FOLIAGE, FLOWERS, AND ROOTS
BLOODROOT (*Sanguinaria*)	ALL PARTS

Plant	Toxic Parts
BLUEBONNET (*Centaurea*)	FOLIAGE AND FLOWERS
BLUE-GREEN ALGAE (*Mycrocystis*)	ALL PARTS
BOSTON IVY (*Hedera*)	ALL PARTS
BOTTLEBRUSH (*Equisetum*)	FLOWER PARTS
BOXWOOD (*Boxus*)	FOLIAGE AND TWIGS
BUCKEYE HORSE CHESTNUT (*Aesculus*)	SPROUTS AND NUTS
BUTTERCUP (*Ranunculus*)	ALL PARTS
CALADIUM	ALL PARTS
CALLA LILY (*Zantedeschia*)	ALL PARTS
CARDINAL FLOWER (*Lobelia*)	ALL PARTS
CAROLINA JESSAMINE (*Gelsemium*)	FOLIAGE, FLOWERS, AND SAP
CASAVA	ROOTS
CASTOR BEAN (*Ricinus*)	UNCOOKED BEANS
CELANDINE (*Chelidonium*)	ALL PARTS
CHALICE; TRUMPET VINE (*Nicotiana*)	ALL PARTS
CHERRY (*Prunus*)	INNER PIT SEEDS
CHINA BERRY TREE (*Melia*)	BERRIES
CHINESE EVERGREEN (*Aglaonema*)	FOLIAGE
CHINESE LANTERN (*Physalis*)	ALL PARTS
CHRISTMAS CACTUS (*Euphorbia*)	ENTIRE PLANT
COLUMBINE (*Aquilegia*)	FOLIAGE, FLOWERS, SEEDS
COMMON PRIVET (*Ligustrum*)	FOLIAGE AND BERRIES
CORAL PLANT (*Euphorbium*)	ALL PARTS
CREEPING CHARLIE (*Glecoma*)	FOLIAGE
CROCUS	BULBS
CROTON	FOLIAGE, SHOOTS
CYCLAMEN	FOLIAGE, STEMS, AND FLOWERS

223

PLANT NAME	TOXIC PORTION(S)
DAFFODIL (*Narcissus*)	BULBS, FOLIAGE, FLOWERS, AND PODS
DAPHNE (*Laurus*)	BERRIES
DEADLY NIGHTSHADE (*Solanum*)	FOLIAGE, UNRIPE FRUIT, SPROUTS
DEATH CAMUS (*Zygadensus*)	ALL PARTS ARE TOXIC; ESP. ROOTS
DELPHINIUM	BULBS, FOLIAGE, FLOWERS, AND SEEDS
DESTROYING ANGEL (DEATH CAP) (*Amanita*; many other fungi)	ALL PARTS OF THE MUSHROOM
DIANTHUS	FOLIAGE, FRUIT
DOGWOOD (*Cornus; Cyboxylon*)	FRUIT MILDLY TOXIC
DUMB CANE (*Dieffenbachia*)	FOLIAGE
EGGPLANT (*Solanum*)	FOLIAGE ONLY
ELDERBERRY (*Sambucus; Alnus*)	LEAVES, BARK, AND SHOOTS
ELEPHANT EAR (TARO) (*Caladium*)	FOLIAGE
ENGLISH IVY (*Hedera*)	ESP. BERRIES
EUPHORBIA (SPURGES)	FOLIAGE, FLOWERS, LATEX-LIKE SAP
FIDDLE LEAF FIG (*Ficus lyrata*)	FOLIAGE, LATEX
FIDDLE NECK (*Senecio*)	ALL PARTS
FIG (*Ficus benjamina*)	FOLIAGE, LATEX
FLY AGARIC DEATH CAP (*Amanita*)	ALL PARTS (CAP AND STEM)
FOUR O'CLOCK (*Mirabilis*)	ALL PARTS
FOXGLOVE (*Digitalis*)	FOLIAGE AND FLOWERS
GELSEMIUM	ALL PARTS
GOLDEN CHAIN (*Laburnum*)	SEEDS AND PODS
GRAPE IVY (*Cissus*)	ALL PARTS
HEART IVY (*Hedera helix*)	ALL PARTS

Plant	Toxic Parts
HEAVENLY BAMBOO (*Nandina*)	ALL PARTS
HEMLOCK ROOTS (WATER & POISON) (*Conium*; *Cicuta*)	ALL PARTS
HENBANE (*Hyoscyamus*)	ALL PARTS
HOLLY, ENGLISH AND AMERICAN (*Ilex*)	FOLIAGE AND BERRIES
HORSE CHESTNUT (*Aesculus*)	ALL PARTS
HORSETAIL REED (*Equisetum*)	ALL PARTS
HYACINTH (*Hyacinthus*)	BULBS, FOLIAGE, AND FLOWERS
HYDRANGEA	ALL PARTS
IMPATIENS (TOUCH-ME-NOT)	ALL PARTS
IRIS (FLAGS)	BULBS AND ROOTS, FOLIAGE, & FLOWERS
IVY (ALL FORMS) (*Hedera*)	FOLIAGE AND FRUIT
JACK-IN-THE-PULPIT (*Arisaema*)	ROOTS ARE MILDLY TOXIC
JASMINE (*Jasminum*; *Gardinia*)	FOLIAGE AND FLOWERS, ESP. NECTAR
JASMINE, STAR *Jasminum*	FOLIAGE, FLOWERS
JERUSALEM CHERRY (*Solanum*)	FOLIAGE AND FRUITS
JESSAMINE	BERRIES
JIMSON WEED (THORN APPLE) (*Datura*)	FOLIAGE, FLOWERS AND PODS
JOHNSON GRASS, WILTED (*Sorgum*)	ALL PARTS
JUNIPER (*Juniperus*)	ALL PARTS
LAMBKILL (SHEEP LAUREL) (*Kalmia*)	FOLIAGE
LANTANA	FOLIAGE, FLOWERS, AND ESP. BERRIES
LARKSPUR (*Delphinium*)	ENTIRE YOUNG PLANT; SEEDS & PODS
LAUREL (*Laurus*)	ALL PARTS ARE TOXIC
LILY OF THE NILE (*Agapanthus*)	ALL PARTS
LILY OF THE VALLEY (*Convallaria*)	FOLIAGE AND FLOWERS
LOBELIA	ALL PARTS

PLANT NAME	TOXIC PORTION(S)
LOCOWEED (*Astragalus; Oxytropis*)	ALL PARTS
LOCUST(S) (*Robinia*)	ALL PARTS
LUPINE (*Lupinus*)	ESP. SEEDS AND PODS, FOLIAGE
MARIJUANA (*Cannabis*)	ALL PARTS
MAY APPLE (*Podophyllum*)	FRUIT
MESCAL (*Lophophora*)	ALL PARTS MAY BE TOXIC
MILK WEED (*Asclepsias*)	FOLIAGE
MISTLETOE (*Viscum; Phorodendron*)	FOLIAGE AND BERRIES
MOCCASIN FLOWER (*Cypripedium*)	FOLIAGE AND FLOWERS
MONKSHOOD (*Aconitum*)	ENTIRE PLANT, INCLUDING ROOTS
MOONSEED (*Menispermum*)	BERRIES
MORNING GLORY (*Ipomoea*)	FOLIAGE, FLOWERS, AND SEEDS
MOUNTAIN LAUREL (*Kalmia*)	YOUNG LEAVES AND SHOOTS
MUSHROOMS (SOME WILD FORMS)	ENTIRE CAP AND STEM
NARCISSUS	BULB, FLOWERS
NECTARINE (INNER SEED ONLY)	ONLY INNER PIT SEEDS
NEPHTHYTIS (*Syngonium*)	FOLIAGE
NICOTINE, TREE, BUSH, (*Nicotiana*)	FLOWERING FOLIAGE AND FLOWERS
NIGHTSHADES (*Solanum*)	ALL PARTS, ESP. UNRIPE FRUITS
OAK TREES (*Quercus*)	LEAVES AND ACORNS
OLEANDER (*Nerium*)	FOLIAGE, STEMS, AND FLOWERS
PANSY (*Viola*)	ALL PARTS
PEACH (*Prunus*)	INNER PIT SEEDS
PEAR (*Pyrus*)	SEEDS (ONLY IF CRUSHED)
PENNYROYAL (*Hedeoma; Mentha*)	FOLIAGE AND FLOWERS

Plant	Toxic Parts
PEONY (*Paeonia*)	FOLIAGE AND FLOWERS
PEPPER (*Piper; Capsicum*)	FOLIAGE
PERIWINKLE (*Vinca*)	ALL PARTS
PHILODENDRON, SOME SPECIES	ALL PARTS
PINKS (*Dianthus*)	ALL PARTS
PLUM (*Prunus*)	INNER SEEDS; FOLIAGE CAN BE TOXIC
POINSETTIA (*Euphorbia*)	FOLIAGE, FLOWERS AND LATEX SAP
POISON HEMLOCK (*Conium*)	FOLIAGE AND SEEDS
POISON IVY (*Tocicodendron*)	FOLIAGE AND FRUIT
POISON OAK (*Rhus*)	FOLIAGE AND FRUIT
POISON SUMAC (*Tocicodendron*)	FOLIAGE AND FRUIT
POKEWOOD OR POKEBERRY (*Phytolacca*)	ROOTS, FRUIT
POPPY (EXCEPT CALIFORNIA) (*Papaver*)	ALL PARTS
POTATO (*Solanum*)	RAW FOLIAGE AND SPROUTS ("EYES")
POTHOS (*Epipremnum*)	ALL PARTS
PRIVET (*Ligustrum*)	BERRIES
PYRACANTHA	FOLIAGE; FRUIT (SOMETIMES)
RANUNCULUS	ALL PARTS
REDWOOD (*Sequoia*)	RESINOIDS LEACHED WHEN WOOD IS WET
RHODODENDRON	FOLIAGE AND FLOWERS
RHUBARB (*Rheum*)	UNCOOKED FOLIAGE AND STEMS
ROSARY BEAN (*Abrus*)	FOLIAGE, FLOWERS, AND PEAPODS
ROSEMARY (*Rosmarinus*)	FOLIAGE IN SOME SPECIES
RUBBER TREE (*Ficus*)	FOLIAGE; LATEX
RUSSIAN THISTLE (*Carduus; Silybum*)	FOLIAGE AND FLOWERING PARTS
SAGE (*Salvia*)	FOLIAGE IN SOME SPECIES
SALMONBERRY (*Rubus*)	FOLIAGE AND FRUIT

PLANT NAME	TOXIC PORTION(S)
SCARLET PIMPERNEL (*Anagallis*)	FOLIAGE, FLOWERS, AND FRUIT
SCOTCH BROOM (*Cytisus*)	LEAVES, FLOWERS, SEEDS
SENECIO ("FIDDLE NECK")	ALL PARTS
SHASTA DAISY (*Chrysanthemum*)	FOLIAGE, FLOWERS
SKUNK CABBAGE (*Symplocarpus*)	ROOTS
SNAPDRAGON (*Antirrhinum*)	FOLIAGE AND FLOWERS
SPANISH BAYONET (*Yucca*)	FOLIAGE AND FLOWERS
SPLIT LEAF PHILODENDRON (*Monstera*)	ALL PARTS
SQUIRREL CORN (*Dicentra*)	FOLIAGE, FLOWERING PARTS, AND SEEDS
STAR OF BETHLEHEM (*Ornithogalum*)	FOLIAGE AND FLOWERING PARTS
STAR THISTLE (*Centaurea*)	ALL PARTS
STRING OF PEARLS (*Seneciao*)	ALL PARTS
SUDAN GRASS, WILTED (*Sorgum*)	ALL PARTS
SUNDEW (*Drosera*)	FOLIAGE
SWEETPEA (*Lathyrus*)	STEMS, SEEDS
TANSY (*Tanacetum*)	FOLIAGE AND FLOWERS
TARO (ELEPHANT EARS) (*Colocasia*)	FOLIAGE
TARWEED (*Eriodictyon*)	FOLIAGE AND SEEDS
TIGER LILY (*Lilium*)	FOLIAGE, FLOWERS, AND SEED PODS
TOAD FLAX (*Linaria*)	FOLIAGE
TOBACCO (*Nicotiana*)	FOLIAGE, FLOWERS
TOMATO PLANT (*Lycopersicon*)	FOLIAGE AND VINES
TOYON BERRY (*Heteromeles*)	BERRIES
TREE OF HEAVEN (*Ailanthus*)	FOLIAGE AND FLOWERING PARTS
TRILLIUM	FOLIAGE

TRUMPET VINE (*Campsis*)	ALL PARTS
TULIP (*Liriodendron*)	BULB, FOLIAGE, AND FLOWERING PARTS
UMBRELLA TREE (*Schefflera*)	ALL PARTS
VENUS FLYTRAP (*Dionaea*)	FOLIAGE AND FUNNEL FLOWERING PARTS
VERBENA	FOLIAGE AND FLOWERS
VETCH (SEVERAL FORMS) (*Vicia*)	SEEDS AND PODS
VIRGINIA CREEPER (*Parthenocissus*)	FOLIAGE AND SEED PODS
WATER HEMLOCK (*Cicuta*)	ROOTS AND FOLIAGE
WILD PARSNIP (*Pastinaca*)	UNDERGROUND ROOTS AND FOLIAGE
WISTARIA (WISTERIA)	FOLIAGE, SEEDS, AND PODS
YELLOW STAR THISTLE (*Centaurea*)	FOLIAGE AND FLOWERING PARTS
YERBA SANTA (*Eriodictyon*)	FOLIAGE AND SEEDS
YEW (*Taxus*)	FOLIAGE

Modified from a list compiled by the *International Turtle and Tortoise Journal* May-June, 1969; a compilation by the San Diego Turtle and Tortoise Society, published in the *Tortuga Gazette* January, 1982; **Poisonous Plants in the Garden**, University of California Agricultural Extension Division; Davis, California; and **MAGIC AND MEDICINE OF PLANTS**, Reader's Digest Association, Inc., Pleasantville, New York; 1986, 464 pp.

APPENDIX C

SPECIES LIST CROSS-REFERENCED BY COMMON NAME

Please note: where a particular species may be known by more than one common name, the other names are listed.

Anchieta's dwarf python	*Python anchietae*
adder; crossed viper; kreuzotter	*Vipera berus*
Aesculapian snake	*Elaphe l. longissima*
African bark or Mopani snake	*Hemirhagerrhis nototaenia*
African beaked snake	*Rhamphiophis multimaculatus*
African burrowing snake	*Chilorhinophis gerardi*
African cape tortoises	*Homopus* sp.
African spotted bush snake	*Philothamnus semivarigatus*
African centipede eating snakes	*Aparallactus* sp.
African cross-barred tree snake	*Dipsadoboa aulica*
African desert mountain adder	*Bitis xeropaga*
African dwarf python	*Python anchietae*
African dwarf wolf snake	*Cryptolycus nanus*
African file snakes	*Mehelya* sp.
African "garter" snakes	*Elapsoidea* sp.
African grass or sand snakes	*Psammophis* sp.
African green snakes	*Philothamnus* sp.
African harlequin snake	*Homoroselaps lateus*
African helmeted turtle	*Pelomedusa subrufa*

APPENDIX C

African house snake	*Lamprophis fulginosus*
African keeled snake	*Pythonodipsas carinata*
African many-spotted reed snake	*Amplorhinus multimaculatus*
African marsh snakes	*Natriciteres* sp.
African mole snake	*Pseudaspis c. cana*
African mountain snake	*Montaspis gilvomaculata*
African quill-snouted snakes	*Xenocalamus* sp.
African rock python	*Python sebae*
African semi-ornate snake	*Meizodon semiornatus*
African serrated star tortoise	*Psammobates occulifera*
African shovel-snout snakes	*Prosymna* sp.
African side-neck turtles	*Pelusios* sp.
African skaapsteker snake	*Psammophylax* sp.
African slug-eating snakes	*Duberria* sp.
African swamp snake	*Limnophis bicolor*
African tent tortoise	*Psammobates tentorius*
African tiger snake	*Telescopus semiannulatus*
African water snakes	*Lycodonomorphus* sp.
African wolf snakes	*Lycophidion* sp.
agama lizards	*Agama* sp.
Aldabra tortoise	*Geochelone (Testudo) gigantea*
alligator, American	*Alligator mississippiensis*;
alligator, Chinese	*Alligator sinensis*
alligator lizards	*Gerrhonotus* sp.; *Elgaria* sp.
alligator snapping turtle	*Macrochelys temminckii*
Amazon River turtles	*Podocnemis* sp.; *Peltocephalus* sp.
amethystine python	*Liasis amethystinus*
Amur viper	*Agkistrodon intermedius*
anaconda	*Eunectes murinus*; *E. notaeus*
Angolan python	*Python anchietae*
anole lizards	*Anolis* sp.
Argentine boa constrictor	*Boa c. occidentalis*
Argentine green speckled snake	*Leimadophis poecilogyrus*
Argentine side neck turtle	*Phrynops hilarii*
Argentine snake-necked turtles	*Hydromedusa tectifera*; *H. maximiliani*

Arizona mountain kingsnake	*Lampropeltis pyromelana*
armadillo lizards	*Cordylus* sp.
Aruba rattlesnake	*Crotalus unicolor*
Asian big tooth snake	*Didodon rufozonatum*
Asian box turtles	*Cuora* sp.
Asian brown tortoise	*Manouria emys*
Asian eyed turtles	*Morenia* sp.
Asiatic keeled box turtle	*Pyxidea mouhotii*
Asian pond turtles	*Heosemys* sp.; *Mauremys* sp.
Asian rat snake	*Gonyosoma oxycephala*
Asiatic roofed turtles	*Kachuga* sp.
asp	*Vipera aspis*
Australia swamp turtle	*Pseudemydura umbrina*
Australian tree snake	*Dendrelaphis punctulatus*
Baja bullsnake	*Pituophis m. vertebralis*
Baja California rattlesnake	*Crotalus enyo*
ball python	*Python regius*
bamboo viper; Chinese tree viper	*Trimeresurus stejnegeri*
banded gecko	*Cyrtodactylus pulchellus*
banded krait	*Bungarus fasciatus*
bandy-bandy snake	*Vermicella annulata*
barba amarilla; fer-de-lance snake	*Bothrops andianus asper*
Barbour's pit viper	*Porthidium (Bothrops) barbouri*
basilisk lizards	*Basiliscus* sp
beaded lizard, Mexican	*Heloderma horridum*
beaked snake	*Rhamphiohis multimaculatus*
bearded dragon lizard	*Pogona vitticeps*; *Amphibolurus barbatus*
bearded lizard	*Amphibolurus barbatus*
beauty snake	*Elaphe taeniua friesi*
Berlander's (Texas) tortoise	*Gopherus (Xerobates) berlandieri*
big-headed turtle	*Platemys megacephalum*
bird snake	*Thelotornis kirtlandii*
Bismark ringed python	*Liasis boa*
black-headed python	*Aspidites melanocephalus*
black-headed snakes	*Tantilla* sp.; *Aparallactus* sp.
black pine snake	*Pituophis m. lodingi*

APPENDIX C

black pond turtle	*Seibenrockiella crassicollis*
black rat snake	*Elaphe obsoleta*
black rattlesnake	*Crotalus viridis cerberus*
black striped snake	*Coniophanes imperalis*
black swamp snake	*Seminatrix p. pygaea*
black-tailed horned pit viper	*Porthidium (Bothrops) melanurus*
black-tailed rattlesnake	*Crotalus molossus*
black tree monitor lizard	*Varanus beccari*
black tree snake	*Thasops jacksoni*
Blanding's turtle	*Emydoidea blandingi*
blind snakes	*Rhamphotyphlops* sp.; *Typhlops* sp.
blood python	*Python curtus*
blue krait	*Bungarus caeruleus sindanus*
blue-striped garter snake	*Thamnophis s. similis*
blue-tongued skinks	*Tiliqua* sp.
blunt-headed tree snake	*Imantodes cenchoa*
boas, common	*Boa constrictor* ssp.
boas, dwarf, Caribbean Island	*Exiliboa, Tropidophis, Ungaliophis*
boa, rainbow	*Epicrates,*
boas, rosy	*Lichanura* sp.
boa, rough-skinned dwarf	*Trachyboa,*
boa, rubber	*Charina bottae*
boa, sand	*Eryx* sp.
boa, tree	*Tropidophis*
Boelen's python	*Liasis boeleni*
bog turtle	*Clemmys muhlenbergi*
Bolson tortoise	*Gopherus (Xerobates) flavomarginata*
boomslang	*Dispholidus typus*
Bornean painted terrapin	*Callagur borneoensis*
box turtle	*Terrapene* sp.
Brahminy River turtle	*Hardella thurjii*
Brazilian smooth snake	*Cyclagras gigas*
brown tree snake	*Boiga irregularis*
brown water python	*Liasis fuscus*
bull snake	*Pituophis melanoleucus* spp.

Burmese mountain tortoise	*Geochelone emys*
Burmese python	*Python molurus bivittatus*
Burmese softshell turtle	*Nilssonia formosa*
bushmaster	*Lachesis muta*
Butler's garter snake	*Thamnophis butleri*
caimans	*Caiman*, sp.; *Melanosuchus niger*
caiman lizard	*Dracaena guianensis*
Calabar burrowing python	*Calabaria reinhardtii*
California kingsnake	*Lampropeltis getula californiae*
Canary Island giant lacerta	*Gallotia stelini*
canebrake rattlesnake	*Crotalus atricaudatus*
Cape cobra	*Naja nivea*
carpet python	*Morelia spilotes variegata*
cascavel, cascabel rattlesnake	*Crotalus durissus*
Caspian turtle	*Mauremys caspica*
cat-eyed snake	*Leptodeira septentrionalis*;
cat-eyed snake; herald snake	*Crotaphopeltis botamboeia*
centipede-eating snakes	*Aparallactus sp.*
Chaco tortoise	*Chelonoides chilensis*
chameleons, old world	*Chamaeleo* sp.; *Brooksia* sp.; *Bradypodion*
checkered gartersnake	*Thamnophis marcianus*
chicken turtle	*Deirochelys reticularia*
Children's python	*Morelia childreni*
Chinese king rat snake	*Elaphe carinata*
Chinese lined rat snake	*Elaphe rufodorsata*
Chinese rat snake	*Elaphe taeniua friezi*
Chinese striped-neck turtle	*Ocadia sinensis*
Chinese tree viper	*Trimeresurus stejnegeri*
Chinese twin spot rat snake	*Elaphe bimaculata*
chondropython	*Chondropython viridis*
chuckwalla lizard	*Sauromalus obesus*; *S. varius*
coachwhip snake	*Masticophis*
cobras	*Aspidelaps lubricus*; *Boulengerina annulata*; *Hemachatus hemachatus*; *Naja* sp; *Pseudohaje goldii*;

APPENDIX C

cobras (*continued*)	*Walterinnesia* sp.; *Ohiophagus hannah*
collared lizards	*Crotaphytus* sp.
scommon garter snake	*Thamnophis sirtalis*
cooter turtles	*Chrysemys* sp.
copperhead rat snake	*Elaphe flavolineata*
copperhead snake	*Agkistrodon contortrix*
coral snakes	*Micrurus* sp.; *Micuroides* sp.; *Maticora birvirgata flaviceps*
crawfish (or swamp) snakes	*Regina* sp.
cribo, yellow-tailed cribo	*Drymarchon c. corais*
crocodiles	*Crocodylus* sp.
crocodile monitor lizard	*Varanus salvadori*
crowned snakes	*Tantilla* sp.
old world smooth crowned snake	*Coronella girondica*
Cuban boa	*Epicrates angulifer*
curly-tailed lizard	*Leiocephalus carinatus*
dab lizard	*Uromastix acanthinurus*; *U. aegypticus*
death adder	*Acanthophis antarcticus*
DeKay's snake	*Storeria dekayi*
desert kingsnake	*Lampropeltis getula splendida*
desert tortoise	*Gopherus (Xerobates) agassizi*
desert viper	*Cerastes cerastes*
diadem snake	*Spalerosophis diadema cliffordi*
diamondback terrapin	*Malaclemys terrapin*
dice snake	*Natix t. tessellata*
dusky rattlesnake	*Crotalus pusillus*
dwarf beaked snake	*Dipsina multimaculata*
dwarf sand adders	*Bitis peringueyi*; *B. schneideri*
dwarf sand lizard	*Eremias grammica*
dwarf tegu	*Calliopistes maculatus*
earless lizards	*Holbrookia* sp.; *Cophosaurus* sp.
earth snake, rough	*Virginia striatula*
earth snake, smooth	*Virginia valeriae*
East African side neck turtles	*Pelusios* sp.
eastern diamondback rattlesnake	*Crotalus adamanteus*

eastern ribbon snake	*Thamnophis s. sauritus*
eastern kingsnake	*Lampropeltis g. getulus*
egg-eating snake	*Dasypeltis scabra; D. atra*
Egyptian tortoise	*Testudo kleinmanni*
elephant trunk snake (or Kurung)	*Acrochordus* sp.
elongated tortoise	*Indotestudo (Geochelone) elongata*
emerald tree boa	*Corallus canina*
Euphrates softshell turtle	*Rafetus euphraticus*
eye lash viper	*Bothriechis (Bothrops) schlegeli*
false coral snakes	*Erythrolamprus bizona; Lampropeltis* sp.
false habu snake	*Macropisthodon rudis*
false map turtle	*Graptemys pseudogeographica*
false water cobra	*Cyclagras gigas*
fat-footed gecko	*Ptyodactylus hasselquistii*
fat-tailed gecko	*Hemitheconyx caudicinctus*
Fea's viper	*Azemiops feae*
fence lizards	*Sceloporus* sp.
fer-de-lance snake	*Bothrops andianus asper*
Fischer's chameleon	*Bradypodion fischeri*
fishing snake; tentacled snake	*Erpeton tentaculum*
flapshell turtles	*Cycloderma* sp.
flat-headed snakes	*Tantilla* sp.
Florida kingsnake	*Lampropeltis getula floridana*
Fly River turtle	*Carettochelys insculpta*
flying gecko	*Ptychozoon kuhli*
flying snakes	*Chrysolopea* sp.
forest cobra	*Naja melanoleuca*
forest racer	*Drymoluber dichrous*
four-eyed day gecko	*Phelsuma quadriocellata*
four-eyed turtle	*Sacalia bealei*
fox snake	*Elaphe vulpina*
frilled dragon lizard	*Chlamydosaurus kingii*
fringe-toed lizards	*Uma* sp.
frog-eyed gecko	*Teratoscincus s. scincus*
Gaboon viper	*Bitis g. gabonica*

APPENDIX C

Galapagos tortoises	*Geochelone elephantopus* ssp.
garter snakes	*Thamnophis* sp.
gavial (gharial)	*Gavialis gangeticus*; *Tomistoma schlegeli*
geckos	*Chondrodactylus* sp.; *Coelonyx* sp.; *Eublepharis* sp.; *Gekko* sp.; *Gehyra* sp.; *Gonatodes* sp.; *Hemidactylus* sp.; *Nephrurus laevis*; *Phelsuma* sp.; *Phyllodactylus* sp.; *Pytodactylus* sp.; *Shaerodactylus* sp.; *Tarentola* sp., etc.
Gila monster	*Heloderma suspectum*
glass "snake" lizard	*Ophiosaurus ventralis*
glossy snake	*Arizona elegans*.
Godman'a pit viper	*Porthidium (Bothrops) godmani*
Gold's tree cobra	*Pseudohaje goldii*
gold thread turtle	*Ocadia sinensis*
gopher snake (bull snake)	*Pituophis melanoleucus* ssp.
gopher tortoise	*Gopherus polyphemus*
grass snakes	*Psammophis* sp.
gray-banded kingsnake	*Lampropeltis mexicana alterna*
gray rat snake	*Elaphe obsoleta spilotes*
Gray's monitor lizard	*Varanus olivaceus* (*V. grayi*)
Great Basin gopher snake	*Pituophis melanoleucus deserticola*
Great Plains gopher snake	*Pituophis melanoleucus deserticola*
Great Plains rat snake	*Elaphe obsoleta emoryi*
Greek tortoise	*Testudo graeca*
green headed tree snake	*Chironius scurrulus*
green night adder	*Causus resimus*
green ratsnake	*Elaphe (Bogertophis) triaspis intermedia*
green snake, rough	*Opheodrys vernalis*
green snake, smooth	*Liopeltis* sp.; *(Liochlorophis vernalis blanchardi)*

green tree monitor lizard	*Varanus praesinus*
green tree python	*Chondropython viridis*
green turtle, marine	*Chelonia mydas*
Greer's kingsnake	*Lampropeltis mexicana greeri*
Günther's garter snake	*Elapsoidea guentheri*
habu snakes	*Trimeresurus* sp.
hawksbill turtle, marine	*Eretmochelys imbricata*
helmeted lizard	*Corythophanes* sp.
herald snake; cat-eyed snake	*Crotaphopeltis botamboeia*
Hermann's tortoise	*Testudo hermanni*
himehabu	*Trimeresurus okinavensis*
hingeback tortoises	*Kinexys* sp.
hog-nosed snakes	*Heterodon platyrhinos* ssp.; *H. nasicus*; *H. simus*; *Lioheterodon madagascariensis*
hog-nosed snake, South American	*Lystrophis* sp.
hog-nosed viper	*Porthidium (Bothrops) nasutus*
hook-nosed snake	*Glyalopion* sp., *Ficimia streckeri*
horned adder	*Bitis caudalis*
horned desert viper	*Cerastes c. cerastes*
hornless desert viper	*Cerastes c. gasperetti; Cerastes vipera*
house gecko	*Hemidactylus garnoti*
iguana, common	*Iguana iguana*
iguana, desert	*Dipsosaurus dorsalis*
iguana, Fiji Island	*Brachylophus* sp.
iguana, ground	*Cyclura* sp.; *Conolophus pallidus*
iguana, marine	*Amblyrhynchus*
iguanas, spiny-tailed	*Ctenosaurus* sp.
impressed tortoise	*Manouria (Geochelone) impressa*
Indian black turtle	*Melanochelys trijuga*
Indian rat snake	*Elaphe helena*
Indian rock python	*Python molurus*
Indian softshell turtles	*Aspideretes* sp.
Indian tree viper	*Trimeresurus gramineus*
indigo snake	*Drymarchon corais* ssp.
Indonesian green water snake	*Enhydris plumbea*

APPENDIX C

Japanese rat snake	*Elaphe climacophora*
jumping viper	*Porthidium (Bothrops) mummifer mexicanum*
jungle runner lizard	*Ameiva ameiva*
Kanburian pit viper	*Trimeresurus kanburiensis*
Kaznakov's viper	*Vipera kaznakovi*
keeled rat snake	*Zaocys dhumnades*
king cobra	*Ophiophagus hannah*
kingsnakes	*Lampropeltis* sp.
Kirtland's bird snake	*Thelotornis kirtlandii*
Kirtland's snake	*Clonophis kirtlandi*
kraits	*Bungarus* sp.
knob-tailed gecko	*Nephrurus laevis*
lacerta lizards, misc.	*Lacerta* sp.
lance-headed rattlesnake	*Crotalus polystictus*
leaf-nosed snake	*Phyllorhynchus decurtatus*
leaf-nosed viper	*Eristocophis macmahoni*
leaf-tailed gecko	*Phelsuma serratocauda*
leaf turtles	*Cyclemys* sp.
leatherback turtle, marine	*Dermochelys coriacea*
legless lizard	*Anniella pulcra*
leopard gecko	*Eublepharis macularius*
leopard lizards	*Crotaphytus collaris* ssp.
leopard tortoise	*Geochelone pardalis* ssp.
lined snake	*Tropidoclonium lineatum*
lined Olympic snake	*Dromophis lineatus*
loggerhead turtle, marine	*Carretta carretta*
long-headed rattlesnake	*Crotalus polystictus*
long-nosed viper	*Vipera ammodytes*
long-tailed brush lizard	*Urosaurus graciosus*
long-tailed rattlesnake	*Crotalus stejnegeri*
Louisiana pine snake	*Pituophis m. ruthveni*
lyre snake	*Trimorphodon biscutatus*
Madagascar big-headed turtle	*Ermynochelys madagascariensis*
Madagascar flat-shelled spider tortoise	*Acinixys planicauda*
mahogany rat snake	*Pseutes poecilonotus polylepis*

Malagasy hognose snake	*Lioheterodon madagascarensis*
Malagasy spider tortoise	*Pyxis arachnoides*
Malagasy tree boa	*Sanzinia madagascariensis*
Malayan flat-shelled turtle	*Notochelys platynota*
Malayan giant turtle	*Orlitia borneensis*
Malayan long-glanded coral snake	*Maticora bivirgata flaviceps*
Malayan pit viper	*Calloselasma rhodosotma*
Malayan snail-eating turtle	*Malayemys subtrijuga*
Malayan soft-shelled turtle	*Dogania subplana*
mambas	*Dendroaspis* sp.
mamushi snake	*Agkistrodon blomhoffi*
mangrove monitor	*Varanus indicus*
mangrove pit viper	*Trimeresurus purpureomaculatus*
mangrove snake	*Boiga dendrophila*
many-banded krait	*Bungarus m. multicinctus*
many-horned adder	*Bitis cornuta*
map turtles	*Graptemys geographica* ssp.
marine (or sea) snakes	*Laticauda* sp.; *Pelamis* sp.
massasaugas	*Sistrusus catenatus* ssp.; *S. ravus*
mata mata turtle	*Chelys fimbriata*
Mediterranean pond turtles	*Mauremys* sp.
Mexican beaded lizard	*Heloderma horridum* ssp.
Mexican giant musk turtles	*Staurotypus* sp.
Mexican green rattlesnake	*Crotalus basiliscus*
Mexican milksnake	*Lampropeltis triangulum annulata*
Mexican moccasin, cantil	*Agkistrodon bilineatus*
Mexican ratsnake	*Elaphe flavirufa*
milksnake	*Lampropeltis triangulum*
Moelendorff's rat snake	*Elaphe moellendorffi*
Mojave rattlesnake	*Crotalus scutulatus*
mole snake, African	*Pseudaspis c. cana*
moloch lizard	*Moloch horridus*
monitor lizards	*Varanus* sp.
Montpellier snake	*Malopon m. monspessulanus*
mountain adder	*Bitis atropos*
mountain horned lizard	*Acanthosaura armata*
mud snake	*Farancia abacura*

APPENDIX C

mud turtles	*Kinosternon* sp.
Muhlenberg's turtle	*Clemmys muhlenbergi*
musk turtles	*Sternotherus* sp.
mussurana	*Clelia clelia*
Namaqua dwarf adder	*Bitis schneideri*
Namib tiger snake	*Telescopus beetzi*
Natal black snake	*Macrelaps microlepidotus*
Natal purple-glossed snake	*Amblyodipsas concolor*
narrow-bridged musk turtle	*Claudius angustatus*
neck-banded snake	*Scaphiodontophis annulatus bondurensis*
New Guinea rat snake	*Elaphe flavolineata*
New Guinea side neck turtle	*Elysea novaguineae*
New Guinea tree boa	*Candoia carinata*
night adders	*Causus* sp.
night lizards	*Xantusia* sp.
night snakes	*Eridiphas* sp.; *Hypsiglena* sp.
Nile monitor lizard	*Varanus niloticus*
Northern Australian Snapping turtle	*Elseya dentata*
northern Pacific rattlesnake	*Crotalus viridis oreganus*
northern pine snake	*Pituophis m. melanoleucus*
olive python	*Python olivaceus*
olive ridley turtle, marine	*Lepidochelys olivacea*
painted turtle	*Chrysemys picta* ssp.
Palestinian viper.	*Vipera palaestinae*
palm vipers	*Bothriechis* (*Bothrops*) sp.
pancake tortoises	*Malacochersus tornei*; *M. procteri*
parrot snakes; flying snakes	*Leptophis ahaetulla*; *L. mexicana*; *Chrysolopea* sp.
patch-nosed snake	*Salvadora hexalepis*
peach throat monitor	*Varanus karlschmidti*
peninsula ribbon snake	*Thamnophis s. sackeni*
Peroni's sea snake	*Acalyptophis peronii*
Philippine rat snake	*Elaphe erythura*
pine snakes	*Pituophis melanoleucus* spp.
pipe snakes	*Cylindrophis* sp.

pit vipers, Asian	*Agkistrodon* sp.; *Calloselasma rhodostoma*; *Deinagkistrodon acutus*; *Trimeresurus* sp.
pit vipers; new world	*Agkistrodon* sp.; *Bothrops* sp.; *Crotalus* sp.; *Lachesis muta*; *Ophryacus undulatus*; *Porthidium* sp.; *Sistrurus* sp.
plated lizards	*Gerrhosaurus* sp.; *Zonosaurus* sp.
pond turtle	*Clemmys* sp.
Pope's tree viper	*Trimeresurus popeorum*
prairie kingsnake	*Lampropeltis calligaster*
prehensile-tail skink	*Corucia zebrata*
Pueblan milksnake	*Lampropeltis triangulum campbelli*
puff adder	*Bitis arietans*
puffing snakes	*Pseutes poecilonotus polylepis*; *P. sulphureus*
pygmy rattlesnake	*Sistrurus miliarius*
queen snake	*Regina septemvittata*
Queensland Fitzroy turtle	*Rheodytes leucops*
racer, blue	*Coluber constrictor* ssp.
racer, Ravergier's	*Haemorrhois ravergieri*
racer, West Indian	*Alsophis vudii picticeps*
racer, yellow-bellied	*Coluber constrictor mormon*
radiated snake	*Elaphe radiata*
radiated tortoise	*Testudo radiata*
rainbow boa	*Epicrates cenchria*
rainbow lizard	*Ameiva ameiva*
rainbow snake	*Farancia e. erythrogramma*
rat (or chicken) snakes	*Elaphe* sp., *(Bogertophis) Spilotes*, sp., *Zaocys dhumnades*
rattlesnakes	*Crotalus* sp.; *Sistrurus* sp.
red-bellied snake	*Storeria occipitomaculata*
red diamond rattlesnake	*Crotalus ruber*
red-eared slider turtle	*Trachemys scripta elegans*
red-footed tortoise	*Geochelone carbonaria*
red milksnake	*Lampropeltis triangulum syspila*

APPENDIX C

red rat snake	*Elaphe g. guttata*
red-necked keelback snake	*Rhabdophis subminiatus*
red-tailed pipe snake	*Cylindrophis rufus*
Reeve's turtle	*Chinemys reevesi*
reticulated python	*Python reticulatus*
rhinoceros viper	*Bitis nasicornis*; *Bitis gabonica rhinoceros*
ribbon snakes	*Thamnophis* sp.
ridge-nosed rattlesnakes	*Crotalus willardi*
ringed sawback turtle	*Graptemys oculifera*
river turtle, Central American	*Dermatemys mawei*
rock lizard, banded	*Petrosaurus mearnsi*
rock rattlesnakes	*Crotalus lepidus* ssp.
rosy boa	*Lichanura trivirgata*
rough necked monitor lizard	*Varanus rudicollis*
rough scaled boa	*Trachyboa boulengeri*
rough scaled sand boa	*Gongylophis conicus*
ruin lizard	*Podarcis sicula*
Russell's viper	*Vipera russelli*
Russian gargoyle lizard	*Phrynocephalus mystaceus*
Russian rat snake	*Elaphe schrenckii*
sage-brush	*Sceloporus* sp.
sail-finned; sail-tailed lizard	*Hydrosaurus* sp.
San Francisco garter snake	*Thamnophis s. tetrataenia*
sand adder	*Vipera ammodytes*
sand boas	*Eryx* sp.
sand "fish" (skink)	*Scincus scincus*
sand lizard (gecko)	*Acanthodactylus pardalis*
sand skink	*Chalcides sexlineatus*
sand snake	*Psammophis* sp.
San Luis Potosi kingsnake	*Lampropeltis m. mexicana*
savannah monitor	*Varanus exanthematicus*
saw scaled viper	*Echis carinatus* ssp.
scarlet kingsnake	*Lampropeltis triangula elapsoides*
scarlet snake	*Cemophora c. coccinea*
sea snakes	*Acalyptophis peronii*; *Aipysurus duboisi*; *A. eydouxi*; *Astrotia*

REPTILE CLINICIAN'S HANDBOOK

sea snakes (*continued*)	*stokesii; Emydocephalus annulatus; Hydrophis* sp.; *Lapemis hardwicki; Laticauda* sp.; *Pelamis platurus*
sharp-nosed viper	*Deinagkistrodon acutus*
sharp-tailed snake	*Stilosoma extenuatum*
sheltopusik lizard	*Ophiosaurus apodus*
shield-nose snake	*Aspidelaps scutatus*
shovel-nosed snake	*Chionactes* sp.
Siamese palm viper; Wirot's pit viper	*Trimeresurus wirotii*
side-blotched lizards	*Uta stansburiana; U. palmeri*
side-necked turtle	*Chelodina longicollis,* etc.
side-striped chameleon	*Chamaeleo lateralis*
sidewinder rattlesnake	*Crotalus cerastes*
Sinai Desert cobra	*Walterinnesia aegyptia*
skinks, large, Australasian, (fruit eating)	*Chalcides* sp.; *Corucia* sp.; *Egernia* sp.; *Mabuya*; sp.; *Tiliqua* sp.; *Trachydosaurus* sp.
skinks, small, insectivorous	*Eumeces* sp.; *Scincella*; sp. *Scincus* sp.; *Lerista* sp.
slider turtles	*Trachemys*
slow "worm" lizard	*Anguis fragilis*
small-headed rattlesnake	*Crotalus intermedius gloydi*
smooth green snake	*Liochlorophis (Opheodrys) vernalis*
smooth scaled water snake	*Enhydris plumbea*
snake eating turtle	*Cuora flavomarginata*
snake neck turtles	*Chelodina* sp.
snail-eating snakes	*Dipsas indica, D.* sp.; *Tropidodipsas sartori*
snapping turtle, alligator	*Macrochelys temminckii*
snapping turtle, common	*Chelydra serpentina*
softshelled turtles	*Amyda cartilagineea; Apalone* sp.; *Aspideretes* sp.; *Chitra* sp.; *Cycloderma* sp.; *Cyclanorbis* sp.; *Dogania sub-*

APPENDIX C

	plana; *Lissemys* sp.; *Palea* sp.; *Pelodiscus*; *Trionyx* sp.
Solomon Island ground boa	*Candoia carinata*; *C. bibroni*
Sonoran gopher snake	*Pituophis melanoleucus affinis*
South African bowsprit tortoise	*Chersina angulata*
South American snake-necked turtles	*Hydromedusa* sp.
South American wood turtle	*Rhinoclemmys punctularia*
Southeast Asian river turtle	*Batagur baska*
southern Pacific rattlesnake	*Crotalus viridis helleri*
southern pine snake	*Pituophis m. mugitus*
speckled kingsnake	*Lampropeltis getula holbrooki*
speckled rattlesnake	*Crotalus mitchelli pyrrhus*
speckled snake, Argentine	*Leimadophis poecilogyrus reticulatus*
spiny lizard	*Sceloporus magister*
spiny neck turtle	*Platemys spixii*
spiny soft-shelled turtle	*Apalone spinifera*
spiny-tailed iguanas	*Ctenosaura pectinata*; *Urocentron*
spiny-tailed lizards	*Uromastix* sp.
spiny turtle	*Geomyda spinosa*
spitting cobra	*Naja n. sputatrix*; *N. nigricollis*
spotted turtle	*Clemmys guttata*
spurred tortoise, African	*Geochelone sulcata*
Sri Lanken pit viper	*Trimeresurus trigonocephalus*
star tortoise	*Testudo elegans*
stinkpot turtle	*Sternotherus odoratus*
Sumatran tree viper	*Trimeresurus sumatranus*
sunbeam snake	*Xenopeltis unicolor*
swifts, Latin American	*Liolaemus* sp.
swifts, North American	*Sceloporus* sp.
Swinhoe's softshell turtle	*Rafetus swinhoei*
taipan snake	*Oxyuranus scutellatus*
Taiwan beauty snake	*Elaphe t. friesi*
Taiwan kukri snake	*Oligodon formosanus*
tegu lizards	*Tupinambis nigropunctatus*; *T. teguixin*; *T. rufescens*

temple turtle	*Heiremys anandalei*
tentacled snake; fishing snake	*Erpeton tentaculum*
tessellated water snake	*Natrix t. tessellatus*
thorny devil lizard	*Heteropterex dilatata*
tic-polonga snake; Russell's viper	*Vipera russelli*
tiger rat snake	*Spilotes pullatus*
tiger rattlesnake	*Crotalus tigris*
tiger snake	*Notechis scutatus*
timber rattlesnake	*Crotalus horridus*
Timor python	*Python timorensis*
toad-headed turtles	*Phrynops* sp.
Tokay gecko	*Gekko gecko*
trans Pecos rat snake	*Bogertophis* (*Elaphe*) *subocularis*
tree lizards	*Urosaurus* sp.
tree snakes	*Abaetulla* (*Dryophis*) sp.; *Imantodes* sp.
tropical chicken (or rat) snake	*Spilotes p. pullatus*
tropical rattlesnake; cascavel cascabel	*Crotalus durissus*
tuatara	*Sphenodon punctatus*
twin-spotted rattlesnake	*Crotalus pricei*
"two headed" snake	*Anilius s. scytale*
two-striped garter snake	*Thamnophis couchi hammondi*
Uracoan rattlesnake	*Crotalus vegrandis*
urutu, wutu snake	*Bothrops alternatus*
veiled chameleon	*Chamaeleo calyptratus*
Vietnamese wood turtle	*Geomyda spengleri*
vine snakes	*Oxybelis* sp.; *Thelotornis* sp.; *Uromacer* sp.
"viper" boa	*Candoia asper*
vipers, old world	*Cerastes*; *Echis*; *Pseudocerastes*; *Vipera* sp., etc.
Wagler's pit viper	*Trimersurus wagleri*
wall gecko	*Tarentola borgetti*
wart snake	*Acrochordus javanicus*; *A. granulosus*
water dragon lizards	*Physignathus* sp.

APPENDIX C

water moccasin	*Agkistrodon piscivorus*
water monitor lizard	*Varanus salvator*
water python	*Liasis olivaceus*
water snakes	*Natrix*; *Nerodia* sp.; *Enhydris* sp.
western ribbon snake	*Thamnophis proximus*
whip-tailed lizard	*Cnemidophorus* sp.
white-lipped forest cobra	*Naja melanoleuca*
white-lipped pit viper	*Trimeresurus albolabris*
white-lipped python	*Liasis albertisi*
wolf snake	*Lycodon aulicus*; *Lycophidion capense*; *L. striatus*
wood turtle	*Clemmys insculpta*
worm snakes	*Typhlops*; *Leptotyphlops*
worm lizards	*Bipes biporus*; *Blanus* sp.
yellow bellied slide turtle	*Trachemys s. scripta*
yellow-footed (legged) tortoise	*Geochelone denticulata*
yellow-headed temple turtle	*Hieremys annandalei*
yellow-lipped (pine woods) snake	*Rhadinaea flavilata*
yellow rat snake	*Elaphe obsoleta quadrivittata*
zebra tailed lizard	*Callisaurus draconoides*

APPENDIX D

SPECIES LIST CROSS-REFERENCED BY SCIENTIFIC NAME

Please note: where a particular species may be known by more than one common name, each name is listed.

Abaetulla (Dryophis) prassinus	Long-nosed tree snake
Acalyptophis peronii	Peroni's sea snake
Acanthodactylus pardalis	sand lizard (gecko)
Acanthosaurus armatus	mountain horned lizard
Acanthrophis antarcticus	death adder
Acinixys planicauda	Madagascar flat-shelled spider tortoise
Acrochordus granulosus	elephant trunk snake; "kurung"
Acrochordus javanicus;	wart snake; "karung"
Agama sp.	agama lizards
Agkistrodon bilineatus	Mexican moccasin, cantil
Agkistrodon blomhoffi	mamushi snake
Agkistrodon contortrix	copperhead snake
Agkistrodon intermedius	Amur viper
Agkistrodon piscivorus	water moccasin snake
Agkistrodon rhodosotma	Malaysian moccasin
Aipysurus duboisi	Dubois's sea snake
Aipysurus sp.	sea snakes
Alligator mississippiensis	American alligator
Alligator sinensis	Chinese alligator

APPENDIX D

Alsophis vudii picticeps	West Indian racer
Amblyodipsas concolor	Natal purple-glossed snake
Amblyrhynchus cristatus	Galapagos Isl. marine iguana
Ameiva ameiva	jungle runner lizard; rainbow lizard
Amphibolurus barbatus	bearded lizard
Amplorhinus multimaculatus	African many-spotted reed snake
Amyda cartilaginea	Asiatic softshell turtle
Anguis fragilis	glass "snake" lizard, slow "worm" lizard
Anilius s. scytale	"two headed" snake
Anniella pulcra	legless lizard
Anolis sp.	anole lizards
Apalone	North American softshelled turtles
Aparallactus sp.	centipede-eating snakes
Arizona elegans	glossy snake
Aspidelaps lubricus	shield nosed "cobra"; Cape coral snake
Aspideretes sp.	Indian softshell turtles
Aspidites melanocephalus	black-headed python
Astrotia stokesii	Stokes's sea snake
Atheris bispidus	Rough-scaled tree viper
Atheris squamiger	bush viper
Azemiops feae	Fea's viper
Basiliscus sp.	basilisk lizards
Batagur baska	Southeast Asian river turtle
Bipes biporus	two-footed worm lizard
Bitis arietans	puff adder
Bitis atropos	mountain adder; berg adder
Bitis caudalis	horned adder
Bitis cornuta	many-horned adder
Bitis g. gabonica; *B. g. rhinoceros*	Gaboon viper
Bitis nasicornis	rhinoceros viper
Bitis peringueyi	dwarf sand adder
Bitis schneideri	Namaqua dwarf adder
Bitis xeropaga	African desert mountain adder
Blanus sp.	two-footed worm lizards

REPTILE CLINICIAN'S HANDBOOK

Boa constrictor ssp.	boa constrictors
Bogertophis subocularis	Trans Pecos rat snake
Bogertophis triaspis intermedia	green rat snake
Boiga dendrophila	mangrove snake
Boiga irregularis	brown tree snake
Bothrops sp.	new world pit vipers other than *Agkistrodon, Bothriechis, Crotalus, Lachesis, Ophryacus, Porthidium,* or *Sistrurus*
Bothrops alternatus	urutu, wutu snake
Bothrops andianus asper	fer-de-lance snake
Bothriechis (Bothrops) schlegeli	eye lash viper
Bothriechis (Bothrops) sp.	palm vipers
Boulengerina annulata;	eastern water cobra
Brachylophus sp.	Fiji Island iguanas
Bradypodion fischeri	Fischer's chameleon
Brooksia sp.	dwarf; stump-tailed chameleons
Bungarus caeruleus sindanus	blue krait
Bungarus fasciatus	banded krait
Bungarus m. multicinctus	many-banded krait
Caiman, sp. *Melanosuchus niger*	caimans
Calabaria reinhardtii	Calabar burrowing python
Callagur borneoensis	Bornean painted terrapin
Calliopistes maculatus	Chilean dwarf tegu lizard
Callisaurus draconoides	zebra-tail lizard
Calloselasma rhodostoma	Malayan pit viper
Candoia aspera	Solomon Island "viper" boa
Candoia bibroni	Solomon Island ground boa
Candoia carinata	New Guinea tree boa
Carettochelys insculpta	Fly River turtle
Carretta carretta	loggerhead turtle, marine
Causus resimus	green night adder
Cemophora c. coccinea	scarlet snake
Cerastes cerastes	desert horned viper
Cerastes c. gasperetti	hornless desert viper
Cerastes vipera	hornless desert viper
Chalcides sexlineatus	sand skink

APPENDIX D

Chalcides sp.	Australasian frugivorous skinks
Chamaeleo bitaeniatus	two-lined chameleon
Chamaeleo brevicornis	short-horned chameleon
Chamaeleo calyptratus	veiled chameleon
Chamaeleo chamaeleon	European chameleon
Chamaeleo cristatus	crested chameleon
Chameleon dilepis	common chameleon
Chamaeleo fülleborni	Fülleborn's chameleon
Chamaeleo gracilis	slender chameleon
Chamaeleo jacksoni	Jackson's chameleon
Chamaeleo johnstoni	Johnston's chameleon
Chamaeleo lateralis	side-striped chameleon
Chamaeleo melleri	Meller's chameleon
Chamaeleo montium	mountain chameleon
Chamaeleo oustaleti	Oustalet's chameleon
Chamaeleo owensi	Owen's chameleon
Chamaeleo pardalis	panther chameleon
Chamaeleo parsoni	Parson's chameleon
Chamaeleo pumilus	dwarf chameleon
Chamaeleo quadricornis	four-horned chameleon
Chamaeleo sengalensis	Senegal chameleon
Chamaeleo sp.	old world chameleons
Chamaeleo tenuis	slender chameleon
Chamaeleo verrucosus	warty chameleon
Chamydosaurus kingii	Australian frilled dragon
Charina bottae	rubber boa
Chelodina longicollis, etc.	long-necked turtles
Chelonia mydas	green sea turtle
Chelonoides chilensis	Chaco tortoise
Chelydra serpentina	common snapping turtle
Chelys fimbriata	mata mata turtle
Chilorhinophis gerardi	African burrowing snake
Chinemys reevesi	Reeve's turtle
Chionactes sp.	shovel-nosed snake
Chironius scurrulus	green headed tree snake
Chitra sp.	Asiatic softshell turtle
Chondrodactylus sp.	geckos

Chondropython viridis	green tree python
Chrysemys picta ssp.	painted turtles
Chrysemys sp.	cooter turtles
Chrysolopea sp.	parrot snakes, flying snakes
Claudius angustatus	narrow-bridged musk turtle
Clelia clelia	mussurana
Clemmys guttata	spotted turtle
Clemmys insculpta	wood turtle
Clemmys muhlenbergi	bog, or Muhlenberg's turtle
Clemmys sp.	pond turtles
Clonophis kirtlandi	Kirtland's snake
Cnemidophorus sp.	race runner, whiptail lizards
Coleonyx sp.	banded geckos
Coluber constrictor ssp.	blue, yellow-bellied racer snakes
Coniophanes imperalis	black-striped snake
Conolophus pallidus	Galapagos land iguana
Corallus canina	emerald tree boa
Cordylus sp.	armadillo lizards; girdled lizard
Coronella girondica	old world smooth crowned snake
Corucia zebrata	prehensile tail skink
Corythophanes sp.	helmeted lizard
Crocodylus sp.	crocodiles
Crotalus sp.	rattlesnakes
Crotalus adamanteus	eastern diamondback rattlesnake
Crotalus atriocaudatus	canebrake rattlesnake
Crotalus atrox	western diamondback rattlesnake
Crotalus cerastes	sidewinder rattlesnake
Crotalus durissus	tropical rattlesnake; cascavel, cascabel;
Crotalus enyo	Baja California rattlesnake
Crotalus horridus	timber rattlesnake
Crotalus intermedius gloydi	Oaxacan small-headed rattlesnake
Crotalus lepidus ssp.	rock rattlesnakes
Crotalus mitchelli pyrrhus	speckled rattlesnake
Crotalus molossus	black-tailed rattlesnake
Crotalus polystictus	lance-headed rattlesnake
Crotalus pricei	twin-spotted rattlesnake

APPENDIX D

Crotalus pusillus	dusky rattlesnake
Crotalus ruber	red diamond rattlesnake
Crotalus scutulatus	Mojave rattlesnake
Crotalus stejnegeri	long-tailed rattlesnake
Crotalus tigris	tiger rattlesnake
Crotalus unicolor	Aruba rattlesnake
Crotalus vegrandis	Uracoan rattlesnake
Crotalus viridis	prairie rattlesnake
Crotalus viridis cerberus	black rattlesnake
Crotalus viridis helleri	southern Pacific rattlesnake
Crotalus viridis lutosus	Great Basin rattlesnake
Crotalus viridis oreganus	northern Pacific rattlesnake
Crotalus willardi	ridge-nosed rattlesnakes
Crotaphopeltis botamboeia	herald snake; cat-eyed snake
Crotaphytus collaris ssp.	collared lizard
Cryptolycus nanus	African dwarf wolf snake
Ctenosaura pectinata	spiny-tailed iguana
Cuora flavomarginata	Asian box turtle; snake-eating turtle
Cyclagras gigas	Brazilian smooth snake; false water cobra
Cyclemys sp.	leaf turtles
Cycloderma sp.	flapshell turtles
Cyclura sp.	rhinoceros iguanas; ground iguanas
Cylindrophis maculatus	spotted pipe snake
Cylindrophis rufus	red-tailed pipe snake
Cyrtodactylus pulchellus	gecko
Dasypeltis atra	egg-eating snake
Dasypeltis scabra	egg-eating snake
Deinagkistrodon acutus	sharp-nosed viper
Deirochelys reticularia	chicken turtle
Dendrelaphis punctulatus	Australian tree snake
Dendroaspis sp.	mamba snakes
Dermatemys mawei	Central American river turtle
Dermochelys coriacea	leatherback turtle, marine
Didodon rufozonatum	Asian big-tooth snake

Dipsadoboa aulica	African cross-barred tree snake
Dipsas indica, D. sp.	snail-eating snakes
Dipsina multimaculata	dwarf beaked snake
Dipsosaurus dorsalis	desert iguana
Dispholidus typus	boomslang snake
Dogania subplana	Malayan soft-shelled turtle
Dracaena guianensis	caiman lizard
Draco volans	flying lizard
Dromophis lineatus	lined Olympic snake
Drymarchon corais ssp.	indigo snake
Drymobius m. margaritiferus	speckeled racer
Drymoluber dichrous	forest racer
Duberria sp.	African slug-eating snakes
Echis carinatus ssp.	rough (saw) scaled sand vipers
Echis sp.	sand vipers
Egernia sp.	spiny-tailed frugivorous skinks
Elaphe sp.	rat (or chicken) snakes
Elaphe bimaculata	Chinese twin-spotted rat snake
Elaphe carinata	Chinese king rat snake
Elaphe climacophora	Japanese rat snake
Elaphe erythura	Philippine rat snake
Elaphe flavirufa	Mexican ratsnake
Elaphe flavolineata	New Guinea rat snake; copper-head rat snake
Elaphe g. guttata	red rat snake; corn snake
Elaphe helena	Indian rat snake
Elaphe l. longissima	Aesculapian snake
Elaphe moellendorffi	Moellendorff's rat snake
Elaphe obsoleta	black rat snake
Elaphe obsoleta emoryi	Great Plains rat snake
Elaphe obsoleta quadrivittata	yellow rat snake
Elaphe obsoleta spilotes	gray rat snake
Elaphe radiata	radiated rat snake
Elaphe rufodorsata	Chinese lined rat snake
Elaphe schrenckii	Russian rat snake
Elaphe (Bogertophis) subocularis	Trans Pecos rat snake

APPENDIX D

Elaphe taeniua friezi	Chinese rat snake; Asian beauty snake
Elaphe (Bogertophis) triaspis intermedia	green ratsnake
Elaphe vulpina	fox snake
Elapsoidea guentheri	Günther's garter snake
Elgaria sp. (*Gerrhonotus*)	alligator lizards
Elseya dentata	North Australian Snapping turtle
Elysea novaguineae	New Guinea side neck turtle
Emydocephalus annulatus	Annulated sea snake
Emydoidea blandingi	Blanding's turtle
Enhydris plumbea	Indonesian green water snake; smooth scaled water snake
Emydura sp.	Australian big-headed side-necked turtles
Epicrates angulifer	Cuban boa
Epicrates cenchria	Brazilian rainbow boa
Eremias grammica	dwarf sand lizard
Eretmochelys imbricata	hawksbill marine turtle
Ergernia sp.	frugivorous skinks
Eridiphas sp.	night snakes
Eristocophis macmahoni	leaf-nosed viper
Ermynochelys madagascariensis	Madagascar big-headed turtle
Erpeton tentaculum	tentacled snake; fishing snake
Erythrolamprus bizona;	false coral snake
Eryx sp.	sand boas
Eublepharus macularius	leopard gecko
Eumeces sp.	insectivorous skinks
Eunectes murinus	anaconda
Eunectes notaeus	yellow anaconda
Exiliboa, Tropidophis, Ungaliophis	dwarf Caribbean boas
Farancia abacura	mud snake; horn snake
Farancia e. erythrogramma	rainbow snake
Ficimia streckeri	hook-nosed snake
Gallotia stelini	Canary Island giant lacerta
Gavialis gangeticus	gavial

Gehyra sp.	geckos
Gekko gecko	Tokay gecko
Geochelone carbonaria	red-footed tortoise
Geochelone denticulata	yellow footed tortoise
Geochelone elephantopus ssp.	Galapagos tortoises
Geochelone elongata	elongated tortoise
Geochelone emys	Burmese mountain tortoise
Geochelone gigantea	Aldabra tortoise
Geochelone (Manouria) impressa	impressed tortoise
Geochelone pardalis ssp.	leopard tortoises
Geochelone sulcata	spurred turtoise
Geomyda spengleri	Vietnamese wood turtle
Geomyda spinosa	spiny turtle
Gerrhonotus sp.; *Elgaria* sp.	alligator lizards
Gerrhosaurus sp.	plated lizards
Glyalopion sp.	hook-nosed snakes
Gonatodes sp.	geckos
Gongylophis conicus	rough-scaled sand boa
Gonyosoma oxycephala	Asian rat snake; mangrove rat snake
Gopherus polyphemus	gopher tortoise
Gopherus (Xerobates) agassizi	desert tortoise
Gopherus (Xerobates) Berlandieri	Texas tortoise
Gopherus flavomarginata	Bolson tortoise
Graptemys geographica ssp.	map turtles
Graptemys oculifera	ringed sawback turtle
Graptemys pseudogeographica	false map turtle
Haemorrhois ravergieri	Ravergier's racer
Hardella thurgi	Brahminy River turtle
Heiremys anandalei	yellow-headed temple turtle
Heloderma horridum	Mexican beaded lizard
Heloderma suspectum	Gila monster lizard
Hemachatus hemachatus;	Ringhal's cobra
Hemidactylus garnoti	house gecko
Hemirhagerrhis nototaenia	African bark snake
Hemitheconyx caudicinctus	fat-tailed gecko
Heosemys sp.	Asian pond turtles

APPENDIX D

Heterodon nasicus	western hog nose snake
Heterodon platyrhinos ssp.	eastern hog-nose snakes
Heterodon simus	southern hog nose snake
Heteropterex dilatata	thorny devil lizard
Homopus sp.	African cape tortoises
Hydromedusa sp.	South American snake-necked turtles
Hydrophis sp.	sea snakes
Holbrookia sp.; *Cophosaurus* sp.	earless lizards
Homoroselaps lateus	African harlequin snake
Hydromedusa sp.	side-necked and snake-necked turtles
Hydrosaurus sp.	sail-tail; sailfin lizard
Hypsiglena sp.	night snake
Iguana iguana	common green iguana
Imantodes cenchoa	blunt-headed tree snake
Indotestudo elongata	elongated tortoise
Kachuga sp.	Asiatic roofed turtles
Kinexys sp.	hingeback tortoise
Kinosternon sp.	mud turtle
Lacerta sp.	lacerta lizards
Lachesis muta	bushmaster snake
Lampropeltis calligaster	prairie kingsnake
Lampropeltis getula californiae	California kingsnake
Lampropeltis g. getula	eastern kingsnake
Lampropeltis getula floridana	Florida kingsnake
Lampropeltis getula holbrooki	speckled kingsnake
Lampropeltis getula splendida	desert kingsnake
Lampropeltis mexicana alterna	gray-banded kingsnake
Lampropeltis mexicana greeri	Greer's kingsnake
Lampropeltis pyromelana	Arizona mountain kingsnake
Lampropeltis triangulum elapsoides	scarlet kingsnake
Lampropeltis triangulum	milksnake
Lampropeltis triangulum annulata	Mexican milksnake
Lampropeltis triangulum syspila	red milksnake
Lamprophis fulginosus	African house snake
Lapemis harwicki	Hardwick's sea snake

Laticauda sp.	Sea snakes
Leadria sp.	armored chameleons
Leimadophis poecilogyrus	Argentine green speckled snake
Leiocephalus carinatus	curly-tailed lizard
Lepidochelys olivacea	olive ridley marine turtle
Leptodeira septentrionalis	cat-eyed snake
Leptophis ahaetulla; *L. mexicana*	parrot snakes
Leptotyphlops sp.	worm snakes
Lerista sp.	insectivorous skinks with reduced limbs
Liasis albertisi	white-lipped python
Liasis amethystinus	amethystine python
Liasis boa	ringed python
Liasis boeleni	Boelen's python
Liasis fuscus	brown water python
Liasis olivaceus	water python
Lichanura trivirgata	rosy boa
Limnophis bicolor	African swamp snake
Liochlorophis vernalis blanchardi	Western smooth green snake
Lioheterodon madagascarensis	Malagasy giant hognose snake
Liolaemus sp.	Latin American swift lizards
Liopeltis sp.	smooth green snakes
Lissemys sp.	Asiatic softshell turtles
Lycodon aulicus	wolf snake
Lycodonomorphus sp.	African water snakes
Lycophidion capense; *L. striatus*	African wolf snakes
Lystrophis sp.	South American hog-nosed snake
Mabuya sp.	frugivorous skinks
Macrelaps microlepidotus	Natal black snake
Macrochelys temminckii	alligator snapping turtle
Macropisthodon rudis	false habu snake
Malaclemys terrapin	diamondback terrapin
Malacochersus tornei	pancake tortoise
Malayemys subtrijuga	Malayan snail-eating turtle
Malocochersus procteri	pancake tortoise
Malopon m. monspessulanus	Montpellier snake
Manouria emys	Asian brown tortoise

APPENDIX D

Manouria impressa	impressed tortoise
Masticophis flagellum ssp.	coachwhip snakes
Maticora bivirgata flaviceps	Malayan long-glanded coral snake
Mauremys sp.	Asian and Mediterranean pond turtles
Mehelya sp.	African file snakes
Meizodon semiornatus	African semi-ornate snake
Melanochelys trijuga	Indian black turtle
Melanosuchus niger	black caiman
Micrurus sp.	eastern coral snakes
Micuroides fulvius	Arizona coral snake
Moloch horridus	moloch lizard
Montaspis gilvomaculata	African mountain snake
Morelia childreni	Children's python
Morelia spilotes variegata	carpet python
Morenia sp.	Asiatic eyed turtles
Naja melanoleuca	white-lipped forest cobra
Naja nigrcollis	spitting cobra
Naja nivea	Cape cobra
Naja sputatrix	spitting cobra
Naja sp.	cobras; also see Aspidelaps lubricus; Boulengerina annulata; Hemachatus hemachatus; Pseudohaje goldii; Walterinnesia sp.; Ophiophagus hannah
Natriciteres sp.	African marsh snakes
Natrix; Nerodia	water snakes
Natrix tessellatus	Dice snake; tessellated water snake
Nephrurus laevis	knob-tailed gecko
Nilssonia formosa	Burmese softshell turtle
Notechis scutatus	tiger snake
Notochelys platynota	Malayan flat-shelled turtle
Ocadia sinensis	Chinese striped-neck turtle
Oligodon formosanus	Taiwan kukri snake
Opheodrys major	Asian smooth green snake
Opheodrys vernalis	rough green snake

Ophiophagus hannah	king cobra
Ophiosaurus apodus	sheltopusik legless lizard
Ophiosaurus ventralis	glass "snake" lizard
Ophryacus undulatus	undulated pit viper
Orlitia borneensis	Malayan giant turtle
Oxybelis sp.	vine snakes
Oxyuranus scutellatus	taipan snake
Pogona vitticeps	bearded dragon lizard
Pelamis sp.	sea snakes
Dogania subplana;	Malayan soft-shelled turtle
Palea steindachneri; Pelochelys bibroni; Pelodiscus	soft-shelled turtles
Pelomedusa subrufa	African helmeted turtle
Peltocephalus sp.	South American River turtles
Pelusios sp.	East African side-neck mud turtles
Petrosaurus mearnsi	banded rock lizard
Phelsuma quadriocellata	four-eyed gecko
Phelsuma serratocauda	leaf-tailed gecko
Philothamnus semivarigatus	African spotted bush snake
Philothamnus sp.	African green snakes
Phrynocephalus mystaceus	Russian gargoyle lizard
Phrynops sp.	toad-headed turtles
Phrynops hilarii	Argentine side-neck turtle
Phyllodactylus sp.	leaf-toed geckos
Phyllorhynchus decurtatus	leaf-nosed snake
Physignathus sp.	water dragon lizards
Pituophis melanoleucus affinis	Sonoran gopher snake
Pituophis m. deppei	Mexican bullsnake
Pituophis melanoleucus deserticola	Great Plains gopher snake
Pituophis m. lodingi	black pine snake
Pituophis m. melanoleucus	northern pine snake
Pituophis m. mugitus	southern pine snake
Pituophis m. ruthveni	Louisiana pine snake
Pituophis m. sayi	bullsnake
Pituophis m. vertbralis	Baja bullsnake
Platemys megacephalum	big-headed turtle

APPENDIX D

Platemys spixii	spiny neck turtle
Podarcis sicula	ruin lizard
Podocnemis sp.	Amazon River turtles
Porthidium (Bothrops) barbouri	Barbour's pit viper
Porthidium mummifer mexicanum	jumping viper
Prosymna sp.	African shovel-snout snakes
Psammobates occulifera	African serrated star tortoise
Psammobates tentorius	African tent tortoise
Psammophis sp.	African sand or grass snakes
Psammophylax sp.	African skaapsteker snake
Pseudapsis c. cana	mole snake, African
Pseudemydura umbrina	Australia swamp turtle
Pseudocerastes	false sand viper
Pseudohaje goldii	Gold's tree cobra
Pseutes poecilonotus polylepis;	mahogany rat snake
Pseutes sulphureus	puffing snakes
Ptychozoon kuhli	flying gecko
Ptyodactylus hasselquistii	fat-footed gecko
Python albertisii	white-lipped python
Python anchietae	Angolan (Anchieta's) dwarf python
Python curtus	blood python
Python molurus	Indian rock python
Python molurus bivittatus	Burmese python
Python olivaceus	olive python
Python regius	ball (regal) python
Python reticulatus	reticulated python
Python sebae	African rock python
Python timorensis	Timor python
Pythonodipsas carinata	African keeled snake
Pytodactylus hasselquistii	fan-footed gecko
Pyxidea mouhotii	Asiatic keeled box turtle
Pyxis arachnoides	Malagasy spider tortoise
Rafetus euphraticus	Euphrates softshell turtle
Rafetus swinhoei	Swinhoe's soft-shell turtle
Regina septemvittata	queen snake
Regina sp.	crawfish snakes; swamp snakes
Rhabdophis subminiatus	Red-necked keelback snake

Rhadinaea flavilata	yellow-lipped (pine woods) snake
Rhamphiohis multimaculatus	African beaked snake
Rhampholeon sp.	Old World chameleon
Rhamphotyphlops sp.	blind snake
Rheodytes leucops	Queensland Fitzroy turtle
Rhinoclemmys sp.	South American wood turtles
Sacalia bealei	four-eyed turtle
Salvadora hexalepis	patch-nosed snake
Sanzinia madagascariensis	Malagasy tree boa
Sauromalus obesus; *S. varius*	chuckwalla lizard
Scaphiodontophis annulatus bondurensis	neck-banded snake
Sceloporus magister	spiny lizard
Sceloporus sp.	fence lizard, swift, sage brush lizards
Scincella sp.	skink
Scincus scincus	sand "fish" skink
Seibenrockiella crassicollis	black pond turtle
Seminatrix p. pygaea	black swamp snake
Sistrusus catenatus ssp.	massasauga rattlesnake
Sistrurus miliarius	pygmy rattlesnake
Sistrurus ravus	Mexican massasauga snakes
Spalerosophis diadema cliffordi	diadem snake
Sphaerodactylus sp.	geckos
Sphenodon punctatus	tuatara
Spilotes pullatus	tropical "tiger" chicken or rat snake
Staurotypus sp.	Mexican giant musk turtles
Sternotherus odoratus	"stinkpot" turtle
Sternotherus sp.	musk turtle
Stilosoma extenuatum	sharp-tailed snake
Storeria dekayi	DeKay's snake
Storeria occipitomaculata	red-bellied snake
Tantilla sp.	black-headed snake; crowned snake; flat-headed snake
Tarentola borgetti	wall gecko
Tarentola sp.	geckos
Telescopus beetzi	Namib tiger snake

APPENDIX D

Telescopus semiannulatus	African tiger snake
Teratoscincus s. scincus	frog-eyed gecko
Terrapene sp.	box turtles
Testudo elegans	star tortoise
Testudo graeca	Greek tortoise
Testudo hermanni	Hermann's tortoise
Testudo kleinmanni	Egyptian tortoise
Testudo radiata	radiated tortoise
Thamnophis sp.	garter snakes, ribbon snakes
Thamnophis butleri	Butler's garter snake
Thamnophis couchi hammondi	two-striped garter snake
Thamnophis marcianus	checkered gartersnake
Thamnophis proximus	western ribbon snake
Thamnophis sirtalis	common garter snake
Thamnophis s. sackeni	peninsula ribbon snake
Thamnophis s. sauritus	eastern ribbon snake
Thamnophis s. similis	blue-striped garter snake
Thamnophis s. tetrataenia	San Francisco garter snake
Thasops jacksoni	black tree snake
Thelotornis kirtlandii	bird snake
Tiliqua sp.	blue-tongued skinks
Tomistoma schlegeli	false gavial
Trachemys s. scripta	yellow-bellied slider turtle
Trachemys scripta elegans	red-eared slider turtle
Trachyboa sp.	rough-skinned dwarf boa
Trachydosaurus sp.	old world frugivorous skinks
Trimeresurus albolabris	white-lipped pit viper
Trimeresurus flavoviridis	habu snake
Trimeresurus gramineus	Indian tree viper
Trimeresurus kanburiensis	Kanburian pit viper
Trimeresurus okinavensis	himehabu snake
Trimeresurus popeorum	Pope's tree viper
Trimeresurus purpureomaculatus	mangrove pit viper
Trimeresurus stejnegeri	Chinese tree viper
Trimeresurus sumatranus	Sumatran tree viper
Trimeresurus trigonocephalus	Sri Lanken pit viper
Trimeresurus wagleri	Wagler's pit viper

Trimeresurus wirotii	Siamese palm viper; Wirot's pit viper
Trimorphodon biscutatus	lyre snake
Trionyx sp.	soft-shelled turtles
Tropidoclonium lineatum	lined snake
Tropidodipsas sartori	snail eating snake, terrestrial
Tropidophis sp.	dwarf tree boa
Tupinambis nigropunctatus;	black and white/yellow tegu lizard
Tupinambis rufescens	red tegu lizard
Tupinambis teguixin	tegu lizard
Typhlops sp.	worm snakes
Uma sp.	fringe-toed lizards
Uromacer sp.	vine snakes
Uromastix acanthinurus;	Bell's dab lizard
Uromastix aegypticus	spiny-tailed lizard
Urosaurus graciosus	long-tailed brush lizard; tree lizard
Uta palmeri	side-blotched lizard
Uta stansburiana	side-blotched lizard
Varanus beccari	black tree monitor lizard
Varanus exanthematicus	savannah monitor lizard
Varanus grayi	Gray's monitor lizard
Varanus indicus	mangrove monitor lizard
Varanus karlschmidti	peach throat monitor lizard
Varanus niloticus	Nile monitor lizard
Varanus olivaceus (V. grayi)	Gray's monitor lizard
Varanus praesinus	green tree monitor lizard
Varanus rudicollis	rough-necked monitor lizard
Varanus salvadori	crocodile monitor lizard
Varanus salvator	water monitor lizard
Vermicella annulata	bandy-bandy snake
Vipera sp.	old world vipers
Vipera ammodytes	long-nosed viper; sand adder
Vipera aspis	asp
Vipera berus	European viper; adder; crossed adder; kreuzotter
Vipera kaznakovi	Kaznakov's viper
Vipera lebetina spp.	blunt-nosed vipers

APPENDIX D

Vipera orsinii	Orsini's viper
Vipera palaestinae	Palestinian viper
Vipera russelli	Russell's viper; "tic-polonga"
Virginia striatula	rough earth snake
Virginia valeriae	smooth earth snake
Walterinnesia aegyptia	Sinai Desert cobra
Xantusia sp.	night lizards
Xenocalamus sp.	African quill-snouted snakes
Xenopeltis unicolor	sunbeam snake
Zaocys dhumnades	keeled ratsnake
Zonosaurus sp.	plated lizards

INDEX

Cryptosporidium 86, 198
Entomelas 87
Giardia 86
Rhabdias 87
Strongyloides stercoralis 87

acepromazine maleate 140, 159
acid-fast staining, for *Cryptosporidium* 86
acid phosphatase, in blood cells 128
acyclovir, dosage of 183
aflatoxicosis due to moldy cricket food 18
alfadolone acetate-alfaxalone acetate 138, 158, 161
alkaline phosphatase, in blood cells 128
amikacin, dosage of 183
aminophylline, dosage of 189
aminosuberic vasotocin, dosage of 179, 189
amoebae, treatment for 197
amoxicillin, dosage of 183
amphoteracin-B, dosage of 189
ampicillin, dosage of 183
amputation, limb 171
anaerobic microbiological culture 89

anesthesia 138–41, 156–59, 161
anophthalmia 15
anophthalmia, in relation to eating 15
anorexia 12
anticoagulants 77
appetite 12
appetite stimulation 192
application of expoxy resin-impregnated fiberglass patches 167
apprehension of prey 20
arginine vascotocin dosage of 179, 189
arthropod ectoparasites, collection and preservation 98
ascorbic acid, dosage of 189
assimilation, of food 25
atropine sulfate, dosage of 189
auscultation 150
autograft, during repair of the chelonian shell 166
autototomy, tail 135
azotemia, determination of 84

bandaging, techniques of 180
barbiturate anesthetics 156–57
basic proteins, in blood cells 129

INDEX

basophils, cytochemical reactions 128–32
benzathine penicillin, dosage of 183
beta carotene 19
beta glucuronidase, in blood cells 128
bicarbonate, plasma 112–17
biopsy, muscle 91–92
blood 73, 78
blood, organic constitutents of 119–25
blood, packed cell volume 119–25
blood anticoagulants 77
blood cell cytochemical reactions 128–32
blood cell histochemistry 131–32
blood cell-specific staining 82
blood collection vial, color code chart 102
blood enzymes, 128
blood film identification 78, 81
blood films, techniques for making 78
blood glucose, determination of 84
blood hemolysis 77
blood staining 80
blood transfusion, heterologous 152
blood transfusion, homologous 152

bone marrow, specimen collection and preparation 79
boredom 22, 23
brain and spinal cord, removal for examination at necropsy 92
brumation 2
buffy coat 78
bunamidine HCl, dosage of 199
buoyancy control via ingestion of stones 24–25

cage heating 9, 28
cage litter material ingestion 23, 28
calcitonin, dosage of 190
calcium glucobionate, dosage of 190
calcium gluconate, dosage of 190
calcium lactate + calcium glycerophosphate, dosage of 190
calcium, plasma 112–17
calcium-phosphorus imbalance 17, 19
calcium:phosphorus ratio 10, 17
calculi, cystic, laboratory analysis 71
carbenicillin disodium, dosage of 184
cardiocentesis 76

INDEX

cardiovascular sounds, abnormal 145–49
carnivory 11
catheter care, 152
caudal alimentary tract specimens 154
cefotaxime, dosage of 184
cell-specific staining 82
cephaloridine, dosage of 184
cephalothin, dosage of 184
cerebrospinal fluid, collection 91
cestodes, treatment for 199
Chelonia (turtles, tortoises, terrapins) 1–2, 53–60
chelonian shell, incision and repair of 165
chemical restraint 137–41, 156–59
chloramphenicol, dosage of 184
chloride, plasma 112–17
chlorpromazine, dosage of 159
choanal slit, swab specimens 153
cimetidine, dosage of 190
clindamycin HCl, dosage 184
clinical methods 133–54
cloacal postovulatory/postcoital plugs 88
cloacal prolapse 161
coccidia, treatment for 197–98
colopexy 163
condom, use for bandaging 180

Crocodilia (alligators, crocodiles, caimans, gharials) 2
cross-polarized illumination for microscopy 86
crushing injury to chelonian shell, evaluation of 170
cryosurgery 171
cryptosporidiosis 86–87
curare 140
cyanocobalamin 191

decalcification of bone-containing specimens 80, 92
decapitation 141
dehydration 151
dental acrylic, use in fracture repair 174
dexamethasone, dosage of 191
diarrhea 27
dichlorvos, dosage of 200
diet, improper 28
dihydrostreptomycin sulfate, dosage of 184
dimethysulfoxide (DMSO), cautionary statement 139, 158
diprenorphine HCl, dosage of 158
dissociative psychotropic agents 138, 157
dithiazine iodide, dosage of 200
dominance, social 8, 28

INDEX

Doppler ultrasonic blood flow detection 77, 145
doxycycline calcium, dosage of 185
drugs, miscellaneous 189
d-tubucurarine, for inducing mydriasis 150
dystocia 179

ectoparasites 72, 202
egg incubation 182
electrocardiography 145
electro-ejaculation 88
electrolytes, plasma 112–17
electronmicroscopy, tissue preparation and fixation 92
elimination 27
embryonic/fetal development, monitoring 149–50
endoparasites 85–87, 197–202
endoparasites, collection and preservation of 98
endothermicity 2
enrofloxacin, dosage of 185
enteropexy 163
enterotomy 162
entromycin, dosage of 191
enucleation, orbital content 164
environmental considerations 7, 28
eosinophils, cytochemical reactions 128–32

epinephrine, contraindication when used with local anesthetics 141
esophageal electrocardiographic probe 145–46
esterase, in blood cells 128
etorphine HCl 158. *See also* diprenorphine dosage and precautions
euthansia 141
exfoliative cytology 91
exploratory celiotomy, chelonian 165
eye, enucleation of 164

febantel, dosage of 199, 201
febendazole, dosage of 201
feces, collection of 85
feces, microscopic examination of 85
feeding frenzy 24
fentanyl-droperidol 157
fermentation, hindgut 22, 162
flatulence 26
fluid, replacement therapy 151–52
flunixin meglumine, dosage of 191
fodder, gathering of 20
food preferences. *See* list of tables
food quality 17
food selection 14
food values 66–69

foreign bodies, gastric, retrieval of 177
fracture repair 161
fungal culture 73
fungal stains 73
furosemide, dosage of 191
furoxone, dosage of 191

gallamine triethiodide, dosage of 156
gas lysis 26
gas production 26
gastric foreign bodies, retrieval of 177
gastric lavage, specimen examination 86–87
gastric lavage, technique for 86
gastrotomy 162
gentamicin sulfate, dosage of 185
gestation times 182
glucose, blood 119–25
glutaradehyde, for fixing tissues for electron microscopy 92
glycophyrrolate, dosage of 191
granulocytes 128–32

halothane 139, 159
heating, cage 11, 26, 28
hemipenial prolapse 161
hemoglobin 119–25
hemolysis 77
herbivory 11
heterologous blood transfusion 152
heterophils, cytochemical reactions 128–32
heterothermia 8
hibernation 2
hindgut fermentation 162
hindgut fermentation by herbivores 22, 162
hindgut processing 22, 162
history, medical 133
Hoyer's mounting medium, for small arthropods 100
humidity 11
hydroxycobalamine 191
hypoglycemia, stress-related, in crocodilians 138
hypothermia for restraint, caution against using 137
hypovitaminosis B_1 17

icterus 83
impaction, intestinal 23, 27
improper diet 28
incision, of the chelonian shell 165
induced mydriasis with d-tubocurarine 150
inhalant anesthetics 139
initial processing of food 23
injection methods 181
insect predation 16

INDEX

intestinal contents, collection for toxicology 96
intestinal impaction 23, 27
intracardiac catheterization 151–52
intracoelomic injection 181
intramedullary infusion of fluid 151
intraosseous infusion of fluid 151–52
intravenous injection 151
isoflurane 139, 159
ivermectin, dosage of 201, 202

Jacobson's organ 15

kanamycin sulfate, dosage of 185
ketamine HCl 138, 157, 161
ketoconazole, dosage of 185

laboratory sample processing 70
lacerations and abrasions, sutureless repair of 176
lactic acid dehydrogenase, in blood cells 128
levamasol HCl, dosage of 200
levamisol phosphate, dosage of 200
lidocaine 140–41
lincomycin, dosage of 185
lingual aplasia 15

lingual aplasia, in relation to eating 15
lipids, in blood cells 129
liquid plastic bandage, use of 164
lithophagy 24–25
local, line, and block anesthesia 161
lysine vasotocin 179, 189

magnesium 19
magnesium, in plasma 112–17
mandibular and maxillofacial fracture, repair of 173
maxillofacial and mandibular fracture, repair of 173
mebendazole, dosage of 201
methischol, dosage of 192
methohexital sodium 157
methoxyflurane 139, 159
metronidazole, dosages of 185, 192, 197
metronidazole, for antibiotic use 192
metronidazole, for appetite stimulation 192
metronidazole, for treatment of amoebiasis 197
microbiological culture, anaerobic 73, 89
microbiological sampling, of respiratory tract 153

microbiology 73
microwave warming, during decalcification of bony specimens 93
microwave warming, of frozen food 18
mineral crystal microscopy 86
mites 72, 202
monitoring, embryonic/fetal development 149–50
monocytes, cytochemical reaction 128–32
motion perception, in relation to eating 15
mounting media, for microscopic specimens 72, 81
mouthpart overgrowth in chelonians, treatment of 176

necropsy 92
nematodes, treatment for 201
nephrotoxic drug administration, precautions for 181
niclosamide, dosage of 199
nitrous oxide 139, 159
nonsurgical retrieval of gastric foreign bodies 177
nontoxic plants suitable for landscaping 219–21
nucleic acids, in blood cells 129
nutrition 10–69
nutritious plants for herbivorous reptiles 63–65

obesity 22, 23
omnivory 11
ophthalmoscopy 150
oral antibiotics, dosages of 183
orbital enucleation 164
orbital venipuncture 75
organic constituents, of blood 119–25
osmotic pressure, of plasma 112–17
osmotic reabsorption of water 14
overcrowding 8, 28
overfeeding 22
overgrown claws in chelonians, treatment of 176
oviductal prolapse 161
oxymorphone 158
oxytetracycline injectable, dosage of 186
oxytocin 179, 192
oxytocin, dosage of 192

pacing behavior, repetitive 22, 176
packed cell volume 119–25
Pampel's fluid for preservation of arthropods and helminths 100
paralyzing agents 140
para-occipital sinus venipuncture 76
parasites, identification of 97–98
parasiticides 197–202

INDEX

parasitological identification 97–98
parenteral antibiotics, dosages of 183–87
paromomycin, dosage of 197
pathology accession form 216–18
pentobarbital sodium, dosage of 156
percussion and auscultation 150
peroxidase, in blood cells 128
pH, of plasma 112–17
phosphorus:calcium imbalance of 17, 19
phosphorus, plasma 112–17
photoperiod 11
physical examination 141
physical restraint 133–38
pica 12
piperacillin, dosage of 186
pituitary, techniques for collection at necropsy 92
plants, toxic 222–29
plasma electrolytes 112–17
poikilothermia 8
polysaccharides, in cells blood 128–29
postoccipital sinus venipuncture 76
postovulatory/postcoital cloacal plugs 88
potassium penicillin G, dosage of 186
potassium, in plasma 112–17

praziquantel, dosage of 199, 201
predatory strike or bite, as a releaser of feeding behavior 24
prednisolone sodium succinate, dosage of 193
preservation of laboratory specimens 72,
prey, quality of 16
prolapse 161, 162
promazine, dosage of 140, 159
pterygopalatine-pharyngeal venipuncture 75
pyrantel pamoate, dosage of 200

radiofrequency electrosurgery 172
ranitidine HCl, dosage of 193
record keeping, by owner 144
rectal prolapse 161
reduced oxygen atmosphere, for anaerobic microbiological culture 89
refuges, in caging 8, 28
repair of the chelonian shell 165
repetitive pacing behavior 22, 176
respiratory tract, obtaining diagnostic specimens of 153
restraint, vago-vagal response, used in 138

retained tertiary spectacle shields, removal of 181
retrieval of gastric foreign bodies 177
Rhynchocephalia (tuatara) 5, 62

salpingotomy/caesarian delivery of impacted ova 164
salt glands 14
salt secretion, extrarenal 14
sample collection 70
Sauria (lizards) 4, 44–52
selection, of food 14
self-induced trauma 23
semen, collection of 88
semen, staining of 89
Serpentes (snakes) 4, 30–43
serum/plasma, abnormal colors of 83
sheared-light microscopy 86
silver sulfadiazine cream 180
simethicone, for relief of intestinal gas 26
social dominance 8, 28
sodium iodide injectable, dosage of 193
sodium, nonrenal excretion of 14
sodium, in plasma 112–17
special bandaging techniques 180
specimen, identification of 78
specimen, preservation of 72
specimen, shipping of 95, 98, 100
splintage of fractures 161
sputum, collection of 87
sputum, examination of 87
Squamata (snakes and lizards) 3
staining, alimentary tract specimens 154
staining, blood and bone marrow 80
staining, feces 85
staining, microbiological specimens 73
staining, protozoa 85–86
staining, respiratory tract specimens 153
staining, sputum 88
staining, urine 84
stains, special, for *Cryptosporidium* and *Giardia* 86
stanzolol, dosage of 193
steatitis, etiology of 17
stethoscopy 145
stomach contents, collection for toxicology 96
stones, consumption of 24–25
stones, formation of. *See* urinary calculi
streptomycin sulfate, dosage of 186
stress 7–8, 24, 28
sucalfate, dosage of 193

INDEX

succinycholine chloride; dosage of 156
sulfadiazine, dosage of 197
sulfadimethoxine, dosage of 186, 198
sulfamerazine, dosage of 197
sulfamethazine, dosage of 186, 198
sulfaquinoxyline, dosage of 186, 198
sulfate, plasma 112–17
surface/area/mass conversions 206
surgical and nonsurgical procedures 160–82
sutureless repair of lacerations and abrasions, 176

tail autototomy, spontaneous, in lizards 135
tapeworms, treatment for 199
teletamine-zolazepam, dosage of 138, 157, 161
temperature conversions 207
temperature, egg incubation 182
temperature, environmental 11, 26
territoriality 8, 12, 28
tertiary spectacle shields, removal of 181
thiabendazole, dosage of 201
thiamin deficiency, food-induced 17
thiaminase 17
thiamylal sodium, dosage of 156
thioglycholate-enhanced microbiological culture 73, 89
thirst 28
ticarcillin, dosage of 187
ticks 72, 202
tincture of benzoin, use in bandaging 180
tissue collection 91
tissue fixation, of brain 92
tissue fixation, of hollow viscus organs 94
tissue fixatives 91
tobramycin, dosage of 187
topical ointments, sprays, and solutions 195
total protein 119–25
toxic plants 222–29
tracheal specimens, collection of 96, 153
tranquilizers, dosages of 140, 159
transcutaneous urocysto-, entero-, and colopexy 163
transport 133–38
transtracheal lavage 153
transtracheal specimens 96, 153
trauma, self-induced 23
trematodes 87
trematodes, treatment for 199, 200

tribromethanol-amylene hydrate, dosage of 158
tricaine methanesulfonate, dosage of 157
trichomonads 87
trichomonads, treatment for 197
trichrome stain, for *Giardia* and other protozoa 85
trimethroprim sulfadiazine, dosage of 187, 198
trimethroprim sulfamethoxazole, dosage of 187
tubocurine 140
turtles, tortoises, and terrapins. *See* Chelonia

ultrasonic Doppler blood flow detection 77
urates 83
urea 119–25
uremia 84
uric acid 119–25
urinary acidification 143
urinary calculi 71, 84
urine, collection of 83
urocystopexy 163

vago-vagal response, induced, use in short-term restraint 138
vapona, dosage of 202
vasotocin 179
venipuncture, sites for 75
venom, effect on preliminary food digestion 24
virological culture, specimen preparation of 90
vitamin A 19
vitamin A, dosage of 193
vitamin B complex, dosage of 193
vitamin C, dosage of 189
vitamin D_3, dosage of 193
vitamin D 19, 20
vitamin K, dosage of 194
vitamin toxicities 19
vomeronasal organ 15
vomeronasal organ, in scent detection 15

water, collection for toxicology 96
water, osmotic reabsorption of 14
water, provision for 13
wound-irrigating solutions 196

xylazine 157